"Every so often a scholar writes a book that has the potential to reshape an academic discipline or at least establish an important new research area or subfield. Elizabeth Hinson-Hasty has done that with this breakthrough Christian ethical engagement with the neglected issue of mental illness. This work has all the hallmarks of great Christian social ethics—it tackles a serious human problem involving profound suffering and injustice, attends to the voices of those most affected, diagnoses societal shortfalls that worsen the problem unnecessarily, brings serious biblical and theological reflection to bear in order to change our moral vision, and offers examples of a path forward for Christian communities. In the end, this is a book that is about far more than *Dutiful Love*. It is about the potentially quite joyful transformation of how all of us relate with individuals and families affected by mental illness."

—David P. Gushee, Distinguished University Professor of Christian Ethics at Mercer University

"A perennial challenge for theologians is to give their work practical import. Elizabeth Hinson-Hasty, a Presbyterian minister and university professor, has written a book that is a superb example of theology that is theoretically and pastorally grounded. She takes her readers beyond thinking about the mere inclusion of persons who suffer from mental illness. She has given us a theology and a blueprint of practices for Christians to adopt in order to give such persons their due, meaning nothing less than their being integral members of their churches and communities."

—Ramón Luzárraga, associate professor and chair of the Department of Religious Studies and Theology at St. Martin's University

"In this perceptive study, Professor Hinson-Hasty recounts the sobering, often sordid, history of social and religious responses to persons with physical and mental disabilities. She then moves beyond that to give voice to individuals and families who confront those realities every day and concludes by calling all of us to nurture and participate in 'communities of caring,' offering creative, insightful ways to do just that."

—Candyce C. Leonard, professor emerita, and Bill J. Leonard, professor of divinity emeritus, at Wake Forest University

"Elizabeth Hinson-Hasty has done something truly remarkable for the field of Christian ethics in this book. Not only has she conducted rigorous research and provided thoughtful analysis, but she also offers a variety of resources to move her intellectual work into the lived experiences of faith communities. This work fills a gap, one known all too well by those of us like her who have siblings with serious mental health conditions."

—Trace Haythorn, executive director of Association for Clinical Pastoral Education

"Elizabeth Hinson-Hasty gifts us with a much-needed, groundbreaking liberation theology for mental health disabilities that speaks the unspeakable: how serious mental illness impacts all of us, including not only the person living with serious mental illness but also their loved ones. This book names important truths about the ways our theological traditions, rituals, and practices disempower people with serious mental illness and their loved ones. Hinson-Hasty faithfully uncovers the stigma and shame that overshadow people living with serious mental illness and their loved ones. This book empowers us to create communities of belonging and to advocate for social change for disabilities and mental health justice."

—Sarah Lund, minister for Disabilities and Mental Health Justice and author of *Blessed Are the Crazy: Breaking the Silence about Mental Illness, Family, and Church*

"Grounded in the vantage point of siblings of those with severe mental illness, *Dutiful Love* offers a sweeping and robust account of Western thought about perceptions of illness and examples of both care and mistreatment. By weaving a rich combination of present-day narratives with biblical, theological, cultural, sociological, medical, and economic analysis, *Dutiful Love* provides a masterful account of Christian responses to mental illness. A theological ethicist, Elizabeth Hinson-Hasty integrates important resources for scholars studying illness, theologians wrestling with suffering, and anyone who cares about how Christian thought and practices shift moral imagination and empower care."

—Heather H. Vacek, vice president and dean of Moravian Theological Seminary and author of *Madness: America Protestant Responses to Mental Illness*

Dutiful
LOVE

11/19/22

MJ-

Enjoy!

Fred

Dutiful
LOVE

*Empowering Individuals and Families
Affected by Mental Illness*

Elizabeth L. Hinson-Hasty

Foreword by Bill Gaventa

FORTRESS PRESS

MINNEAPOLIS

DUTIFUL LOVE
Empowering Individuals and Families Affected by Mental Illness

Cover design: John M. Lucas
Cover images: Markus Spiske @ Unsplash

Print ISBN: 978-1-5064-6488-6
eBook ISBN: 978-1-5064-6489-3

Dedicated to Kelly Clark Kunze and Pamela Ruth Prouty
two friends who model inclusion and
nurture communities of belonging

Contents

Additional Resources

Foreword

Brothers and Sisters in the Faith:

People involved in Christian faith communities of many types love to use the language of families. We talk about "the family of God," a "church family," a "church father," a "mother of the church," "children of God," our "extended church family," being "welcomed into the family," and "belonging to our church family." Some Christian traditions use "Brother" and "Sister" as the titles of ordained clergy or members of religious orders. Others also use that terminology for lay leadership in the church such as deacons or others who are simply respected for their longtime relationship with and service to a congregation. At other times, we simply talk about our "brothers and sisters in faith." These family metaphors, images, and titles all convey respect for long-term relationships that guide, sustain, and support members of the faith community and one another.

They also speak to our hope and commitment to love one another as a family, but as we all know, both church families and biological families are not always seas of calm for smooth sailing. Storms and rough patches can come from within and without. There are times when individual issues impede the capacity to function as a family unit; other times, the rest of the family have to carry the responsibilities of another to sustain day-to-day life and keep a family together. Sometimes, others are called to take over until a family member is able to pick up their role again. But that is all part of what it means to belong to a family, to be a home that is also sanctuary, where the "ties that bind" nourish and sustain all of us in the wider world. Both families and churches, we hope, are places where "everybody knows our names" and we are known well—places we can go where they "gotta take us in" because that's just what we are supposed to do.

In the last few decades, more and more attention has been paid to members of both church and natural families who have to deal with challenges that are neither temporary nor easily fixable. These include multiple forms of disabilities that need more than typical levels of support. Thankfully, there has been an ever-growing awareness of families with children and/or adult members with physical and/or intellectual disabilities in educational, community, and congregational settings. We have moved from the development of inclusive public education programs to inclusive religious education programs, from public systems and advocacy groups that provide some family support to an ever-greater awareness of the ways that churches can support all the members of biological families as well as the individuals with disabilities. We are learning about the redemptive power of welcome and support when all members of a family are included as well as about the wounding pain and isolation when they are not. Paraphrasing Matthew 25:40, "As we do unto people with disabilities (often seen as the least of these) and their families, so we do it unto our Lord."

While congregations are paying more attention to families with members with various forms of disabilities, many faith communities are just beginning to recognize the prevalence of mental health issues in society and perhaps in their midst. Individuals dealing with mental illness and their family members often experience a hellacious journey even in the best of circumstances. Finding appropriate and effective care is one thing; sustaining that care over the long haul is another. Mental illness is not something that is easily fixed or controlled. The common perception is that since mental illness is neither an intellectual nor physical disability, the right attitude or a bit more willpower should take care of it. That is simply another version of "If your faith was strong enough, you could be healed," an injunction that adds the diagnosis of lack of faith to a chronic condition when that cure does not happen.

Another concern is that while inclusive and supportive ministries in congregations have frequently addressed the needs of parents over the long haul, little attention has been paid to siblings. Disabilities can isolate individuals and families, including siblings. Siblings often take on major roles in supporting a brother or sister in both recognized and unrecognized ways. Caring for one's brother or sister is a typical part of healthy family life, but extra roles, and the isolation caused by the attitudes of others compound those roles for siblings, particularly when they may have to assume additional caregiving responsibilities as their parents age.

In this book, Elizabeth Hinson-Hasty focuses on mental illness and the potential response of faith communities through the particular perspective of brothers and sisters who live with or provide support for siblings affected by mental illness. It is this third focus that makes this book a unique contribution. Congregations can support individuals with disabilities in various ways, including those with mental illness, but it is critical that support is sustained over the long haul. This means walking alongside those who support and provide primary care for people with mental illness. In most cases, these caregivers are immediate family and sometimes grandparents and other relatives.

To support a person with mental illness and those who care for them, we should begin by asking, How would we welcome and include anyone? Help does not need to start as a program. Forms of support may rise organically from those relationships that can match needs with the gifts and strengths of others in the congregation. Pastors making accommodations to enable inclusion in worship and friends and staff who listen, provide respite, stay in touch, invite participation, and offer ways for an individual and their family members to contribute to the life of a congregation are some of the ways faith communities are responding.

Simply having a congregation learn about and reflect on mental illness is one major step. One of my favorite stories is from a pastor who said that after he included prayers for people with mental illness and their families in the Sunday morning pastoral prayer for the first time, his phone did not stop ringing on Monday. Why? People now knew it was safe to call him and that they could bring their personal and spiritual journeys related to mental illness into the sanctuary of pastoral and congregational care.

When we support the individuals with mental illness and their primary caregivers, we must remember that they may be in the midst of a long search for appropriate forms of care in the wider community. Support may be needed from various sources: mental health professionals, education systems, potential employers, and due to the dearth of effective mental health services in many communities, sometimes the police, because a *small* percentage of people with mental illness may exhibit problematic behaviors in public settings, often as a cry for help. Professionals in mental health can do things congregations and friends cannot, but the reverse is also true. Congregational friends and advocates can help find those supports and, as appropriate, collaborate with them in developing a community network of care. An African proverb uses the wonderful metaphor of the whole body in saying that "when a thorn is stuck in the foot, the whole body must stoop to pluck it out."

If we think mental illness is sometimes confusing and mysterious, the same labels apply to public services and systems of care. Where do we find them? How do we get through the hoops of eligibility? Does insurance pay for help? How do we understand the acronyms and language that seem normal to people who work in those services but not to anyone else? The questions, one might say, are legion, like the spirits thought to inhabit the man Jesus met in the tombs in the country of the Gadarenes (Matthew 8:28–34). They sometimes don't make sense either.

Part of ministry means learning how to be effective in what can seem like a strange and foreign world. To do that, we have to deal with cultural, religious, and social attitudes, beliefs, and practices that have arisen over centuries of dealing with human beings affected by mental illness. History is filled with outdated ideas, superstitions, abandoned methodologies of care, stigmas that associate mental illness with all kinds of mythical or spiritual forces, and multiple forms of media and other public discourse that focus on the most unusual instances or the most insidious forms of stereotypes. It also means dealing with an all-too-frequent outcome of mental illness: poverty. The church has had a role in all of this, which means that in order to undertake new journeys of support and accompaniment, much unpacking must be done. One of the valuable and necessary ways congregations can support individuals is to address the unhelpful attitudes, stereotypes, and systems that surround disability. This is a crucial first step in empowering both the congregation and the persons whose lives are impacted by disability. Addressing these stereotypes is a clear signal of a congregation's intention to stand with people as they live with mental illness and seek avenues of treatment and recovery.

This can take the form of learning about mental illness and those sys-tems of care, educating about the history of attitudes and stereotypes, and reinterpreting Scriptures that have been used to create or justify unloving behavior. It can be refusing to let labels define a person or family, because the primary labels that matter are "child of God" and "member of the body of Christ." It means recognizing, as the famous TED talk by Chimamanda Ngozi Adichie says, "the danger of a single story" and making sure we see that every person is a bundle of stories, passions, interests, and gifts—in addition to needs. Empowerment begins with knowing you do not stand abandoned or alone and that others know your name and your stories.

We in the church also love to talk about our public witness to the love of God and the power of faith. An incredible act of witness is rallying around the person with mental illness and with those closest to them. This means including them and standing with them as they find their way in a world that does not understand and is sometimes hostile. This visible support is a witness to the individual and family; to their friends, colleagues, and wider family; and to those who work in mental health services who often despair of helping clients find what they have no power to give. It is also a witness to all of the members of the church family and other faith communities. Like a beautiful stone thrown into a pond, the ripples go out in all directions. We also call that evangelism.

So gear up, church family, and help individuals with mental illness, their parents, and their siblings prepare for what can be a long journey. Sustaining the family of believers so that we each respond to God's call has been what the church has always been about. We are all brothers and sisters in Christ.

Bill Gaventa
Author, educator
Founder of the Institute on Theology and Disability

Acknowledgments

Before I give thanks for the many people who helped me in the process of writing this book, I want to acknowledge the fact that this is the first book I have written during a pandemic. Social distancing measures and the quick move to online teaching forced me to become a multitasker like never before. I ask for some generosity from readers if there are deficiencies in this text due to that circumstance. At the same time, I want to suggest that the challenges we all faced during the pandemic provide further evidence of the book's importance. The COVID-19 pandemic reminded all of us of our deep connection as human beings and underscored social inequalities and the way our society too often fails to provide social safety nets to support families in times of tumult and transition.

My ultimate hope in writing these pages is to join a journey with other siblings who have brothers and sisters struggling with mental health issues and to share what I have learned about why the obstacles to creating the basic conditions necessary for their family members to survive, thrive, and flourish are so great and difficult to climb over. Due to the silence surrounding serious mental illness in my family, the circumstances of my mother's death forced me to become a quick study. When I started talking about the caregiving responsibilities that I would take on and sharing the challenges ahead, friends began to share their stories too. However, the greatest compliment and encouragement I received throughout the process of writing this book came from my brother when he began to be more open with me and identify me as "a helper." Sharing stories with others did much more than make me feel better; these stories became an invisible but tangible web of empowerment, wisdom, and hope.

I want to express my deep gratitude to all those who helped me with this project along the way by providing funding for a sabbatical, participating in an interview, listening to my ideas while they were forming, or reading drafts of chapters. There are many who need to be named. Bellarmine University generously granted my request to take a yearlong sabbatical and supported me in the process of seeking siblings whom I could interview. The Louisville Institute graciously awarded me with a Sabbatical Grant for Researchers that provided the financial support I needed to devote myself to this project. I participated in the Winter Seminar sponsored by the Louisville Institute and was greatly inspired by members of my small group, who represented a variety of disciplines, affirmed my vision for the work, and challenged me with their constructive comments to think in new directions.

Several friends, colleagues, and mental health advocates read my first proposal for the Louisville Institute grant, commented and offered corrections to drafts of chapters, listened and brainstormed with me, or took long walks and shared ideas as I was thinking through this project. I would be remiss if I did not publicly thank Scott Tunseth and the editorial team at Fortress Press, Dean Bucalos, Georgine Buckwalter, Burton Cooper, James Calvin Davis, Elizabeth Dinkins, Mark Douglas, Bill Gaventa, Roger Gench, Trace Haythorn, Jessica Hume, Katherine Johnson, Bill Leonard, Ellen Ott Marshall, JoAnne Morris, Shelby Nodler, Francesca Nuzzolese, Doug Ottati, Annette Harris Powell, and Sheila Schuster. Mental health advocates have been particularly helpful in the process of writing because they have pressed me to recognize that in a project such as this, people are the primary "texts" and sources of knowledge, and their stories are the ground and center of theological reflection. My colleagues in the Department of Theology at Bellarmine University—Hoon Choi, Joseph Flipper, Greg Hillis, Justin Klassen, and Deborah Prince—are also an ever-present source of encouragement, friendship, generative dialogue, and strength. They had to take on new tasks in order for me to take a year away from teaching at the university, and I deeply appreciate their time and support. Finally, I am always exceedingly grateful to Lee, Garrison, and Emmeline Hinson-Hasty, my family, who live this journey with me, listen even when they get tired, and prop me up or help me find humor and fun on some of the most chaotic days.

Introduction

Love puts up with all things,
trusts in all things,
hopes for all things,
endures all things.
Love never fails.

—1 Corinthians 13:7–8

Dutiful love greeted me in my brother's voice when I answered my cell phone shortly after midnight on a Thursday morning. My mother had fallen earlier in the day, and by evening, Chris noticed a knot swelling on the back of her head. He thought she ought to go to the hospital for medical attention. Dementia and other medical conditions took over the last five years of my mother's life. I was the first person my brother would call after the ambulance arrived at my parent's home. On that early morning, Chris asked me to meet my mother and father in the emergency room. It is not that I minded going to meet them. There was never a question in my mind when I picked up the phone about whether it was my duty to go. Of course, I loved my mom. She gave birth to me and raised me. She was there for me on more occasions than I can count. She picked up the phone to share recipes, to just talk, or after I married and had my own children, to give me advice about how to handle their needs. Nevertheless, it was the middle of a busy week at work, and my daughter had a project due the next day, which required me to be present at her school later in the afternoon. The thought of waiting for hours in the emergency room came with some dread, especially knowing the exhaustion factor for the day ahead. Fortunately, I had a job that would understand if I needed to be late the next morning. Still, you can imagine the energy I had to muster to pull on my clothes again. I would not have described my feelings at that moment with the sentiment worthy of an emotion like love, but love has many meanings.

It is impossible to settle on a single definition of love no matter how hard we try in popular conversations and in theological writings. Love is complex because people and relationships are complicated. We all live in such varied circumstances. Loving others isn't always tied to emotions. Love also has a dimension that transcends human understanding and escapes the limits of human language. Philosophers and theologians write about self-love, neighbor love, romantic love, affectionate love, steadfast love, obsessive love, familial love, playful love, self-sacrificial love, self-giving love, and love shown by being present. In these pages, I will invite you to reflect with me on self-sacrificial (kenotic) love as it is framed by Christian faith and to consider self-giving love as an alternative way of living out dutiful love, particularly as caregivers.

My story is not unique. There are presently about 43.5 million other adults in the United States providing unpaid care for another adult or child who is living out a similar story in different places and spaces.[1] Caregiving is stressful, demands multitasking, and makes a life-sustaining contribution both socially and financially to people whom we love. Being present during times of sickness, whether periodic or chronic, is one of the ways that we expect our family, faith communities, and close friends to show their love for us because of the ties that bind us together. When researchers asked a group of caregivers about what made them take on the responsibility of caregiving, over half said they felt they have no other choice but to do so.[2] Dutiful love motivated them, and it motivated me.

You may have wondered when you began reading why I was the one called to go to the hospital that morning. One part of my story that not all caregivers will share is the serious mental illness that affects my family. My father, E. Glenn Hinson, has written openly in his memoir *A Miracle of Grace* about my brother's serious mental illness. However, he offers little reflection on its impact on me as a sibling or the way our society uses disability to define a social identity and to discriminate against people with mental and physical impairments. Family members attend to each other's needs within a much larger context—social, economic, political. There is a certain order of relationships that our society enforces by associating the most fully able bodies and minds with the "normal," and this imposed order shapes the realities of people with disabilities and their entire family system. These conditions often require siblings to deny their own needs in order to provide space for their parents to care for someone struggling with anxiety, debilitating depression, or episodes of mania.

My experience growing up in a family affected by serious mental illness and now as a caregiver raises significant questions for me as a sibling and a scholar of theology and ethics about the connection between self-sacrificial, dutiful love and caregiving in Christian thought and practice. What about when that dutiful love and the call to self-sacrifice extend over the course of an entire lifetime because of social limitations placed on a person due to chronic physical or mental illness? What about the ways dutiful love and the call to self-sacrifice influence more than one individual life and shape an entire family system, maybe even a larger community? How should Christians tell the story of Jesus living for and laying down his life for others within a larger social, economic, and political context in which concepts of normal and abnormal, able bodied and disabled function in ways that mark and define individual identities and the roles they take on within their families?

One publication of the National Alliance on Mental Illness (NAMI) written to help siblings and offspring of people with mental illness deal with their feelings suggests that we "carry a legacy that permeates the crawl spaces of [our] adult lives. That legacy has personal, interpersonal, occupational, and family components."[3] I can personally give testimony to the truth in the legacy left for siblings. For the last ten years of my mother's life, I felt like a bystander looking on at her relationship with my brother from a distance. On the surface, I was not needy enough to be let into their relationship. Often, my needs and those of my children were neglected because there were other events in their household demanding urgent attention. I felt both forgotten and guilty that I needed more time and attention.

We did not speak too much about mental illness among ourselves or with others except in terms of visits to doctors and therapists and picking up medications at the local pharmacy. Some of this had to do with the fact that no one in my family had the time, energy, or access to resources to examine carefully our society's understanding of mental disability and to challenge the way it shaped our lives together as mother, father, brother, and sister. Much of this had to do with the stigma and shame associated with mental illness. Stigma is a heavy burden that our society places on individuals and families affected by serious mental illness. We had to put on a public face that would be acceptable to others. I also don't think people always know how to respond when you do risk disclosing the truth. Thus for several years, I just avoided telling others, but that decision came with a feeling of profound isolation, a strangeness and estrangement that impacts all of my relationships.

It wasn't until my mother's death and I was called on to be the caregiver that I became aware that other friends and family members knew about my brother's serious mental illness. In the last weeks of my mother's life, I began sharing more openly with friends some of the challenges we were facing as a family and discovered that no one was surprised. Many others were quite aware of the situation. Some offered to help find housing for my brother even though that need had existed for quite some time. There was no good news in that news. Community relationships and social bonds weave together into an indispensable and irreplaceable fabric of care. However, these relationships and social bonds all too often break down when you factor in serious mental illness. My newfound awareness gave me a longing to confront the stigma and silence surrounding the impact of my brother's condition on my family and to examine more carefully the larger context in which we are making decisions about caring for each other's needs. More so, that awareness compelled me to enter into the crawl spaces of my household in an effort to find a more life-giving and empowering way to connect dutiful love and caregiving.

Dutiful Love and Self-Sacrifice as Defined by the Christian Tradition

Dutiful love puts up with and endures all things for the sake of another's needs; it demands that we make sacrifices because others need us. Love, compassion, and caregiving are important concepts in many religious traditions, though they may not be interpreted in exactly the same way. The central act of the Christian narrative is Jesus laying down his life for the sake of others. There is no way for Christians to avoid this part of the story no matter how counterintuitive it may seem in Western consumer societies. It doesn't matter how you name your own social identity or the theological world with which you identify; the Christian year always culminates in Jesus heading to the cross, where he empties himself of all of his embodied power. Jesus's self-sacrifice is not an end in itself or the end of the story. Paul reflects on Jesus's sacrificial act in his letter to the Philippian community of faith as he writes, "But he emptied himself by taking the form of a slave and by becoming like human beings. When he found himself in the form of a human, he humbled himself by becoming obedient to the point of death, even death on a cross" (Philippians 2:7–8). Jesus's unselfish act embraces the fullness of our humanity. Christ's death on the cross reveals the depth and vulnerability of God's suffering love for us.

For centuries, Christian theologians have equated divinity with unselfish love. Reformed theologian Jürgen Moltmann writes, "God is unselfish love. Kenosis is the mystery of the trinitarian God. By virtue of God's unselfish love, God permeates all creatures and makes them alive. In this way God loves in the creation community and allows the community of all God's creatures to live in God. . . . The unselfish empathy of God awakens the sympathy of all creatures for each other."[4]

Living in God invokes empathy and invites self-sacrifice—love overflowing from one body to the next in a never-ending, ever-creating cycle. Egocentrism, independence, self-centeredness, greed, and the inability to surrender or compromise one's own goals and needs for another's sake are the enemies of self-sacrificial and dutiful love.

Stories and Theories to Help Us Understand the Context of Self-Sacrifice and Dutiful Love

Although many Christian theologians have praised kenosis as a beautiful ideal, self-sacrifice is a very troubling concept even in the abstract. The notion of self-sacrifice within such an individualistic and market-oriented society as the United States is inherently tied to a loss of self and community. Discussions examining the relationship of individual needs to a larger common good are easy to avoid in this context. There are many individual caregivers who want to help their family members or serve others in society, but their care for others comes at the expense of realizing their own dreams and attending to their own needs, health, and well-being. Studies show that choice is "an important aspect of caregiving."[5] Without choice, caregivers can increase their own vulnerabilities.

A larger context of economic, social, and political power relations forms our understanding and practice of dutiful love and caregiving. I am not the first feminist theological ethicist to point out that Christian communities of faith too often fail to confront the attitudes, systems, and structures that privilege some people, communities, and nations over other social groups and the needs of the planet as a whole.[6] Idealized norms of self-sacrifice and dutiful love neglect the way in which our society promotes caregiving for more privileged individuals and social groups at the expense of the needs of others who have less privilege, money, and power. The truth is that our humanity depends on reciprocity—other people and the planet giving to us and us giving to others. What we need is a way of articulating an understanding of self-sacrificial and dutiful love that is life-sustaining and provisioning for all.

Ellen Ott Marshall relates what it felt like to live out "self-sacrificial" or "dutiful love" during pregnancy. Marshall is an ethicist, a mother, a wife, a daughter, a professor, and a religious leader in the United Methodist Church. When she was pregnant with twins, her doctor prescribed bed rest for a number of weeks. You can imagine that halting her many commitments came as a great challenge and annoyance. Marshall remembers feelings of anxiety, boredom, and isolation, none of which comes first to mind when thinking about love. A friend praised her for embodying "the paradigmatic act of love"—the kind of love Christian tradition has taught us will make sacrifices, even if it means giving up one's own life for others. "Like many women," Marshall observes, "I have been shaped by the idea that we demonstrate the depth of our love by the extent of our giving."[7] However, she also admits that bed rest did not make her feel worthy of praise. Instead, she felt "ugly and uncomfortable, resentful and anxious, occasionally depressed and angry, and terribly sensitive."[8] An extended period of hospitalization near the end of her pregnancy left Marshall feeling "stripped of personhood" as she rested for a week in a nondescript hospital gown while nurses and doctors attended to her and the twins' needs. Ultimately, Marshall learned from her experience that while sacrificing herself to care for the twins still gestating in her womb was a source of deep joy and fulfillment, it also left her feeling depleted. She needed what she called "life-restoring love" to balance her sacrifices.

Overly romanticized notions of the "good family" can powerfully inform and shape the imperative for mothers in the Christian faith to live out self-sacrificial love. Mary all too often is lifted up as a model for her willingness to submit to a divine command to bring Christ into the world without our reflecting on the contemporary context in which women are living within families and whether or not the larger society has established the conditions necessary to sustain family life, particularly for those with chronic health issues. Women report higher levels of guilt when they are unable to take on the burden of care, are forced to limit their own responsibilities for caregiving, and/or unable to control the outcomes for those whom they are responsible.[9]

Valerie Saiving's 1960 article "The Human Situation: A Feminine View" provides an earlier example of the feminist questioning of self-sacrificial love and male theologians' failure to incorporate the reality of women's experiences into their theories.[10] Feminist theologians reject theories offered by men in power that keep women in powerless, subservient roles. Daphne Hampson, a post-Christian theologian, and Sarah Coakley, a Christian systematic theologian, continued the early debate by focusing specifically on developing feminist responses to idealized notions of kenosis, or self-sacrificial love. For Hampson, *self-sacrifice* is synonymous with *powerlessness* and *self-effacement*. Coakley argues that when paired with contemplation, self-sacrifice can embody power and empowerment in vulnerability.

Womanist scholars add another perspective by confronting white feminist theologians for defining women's experiences too narrowly as they unpack a racialized social, economic, and political context in which

Christians talk about and embody self-sacrificial love. Cheryl Townsend Gilkes calls out the cultural humiliation of Black women's bodies in white supremacist societies. The commodification of Black women's bodies that began with slavery continues through culturally established ideal norms for beauty in whiteness, the hypersexualization of Black women's bodies, and pervasive stereotypes such as mammies who appear to be content to serve white needs. Gilkes points to the poet Alice Walker's definition of *womanist* as a way to name resistance: "Loves music. Loves dance. Loves the moon. Loves the Spirit. Loves love and food and roundness. Loves struggle. Loves the Folk. Loves herself. *Regardless*."[11] Love in Walker's words resists cultural humiliation as it embraces loving oneself, *regardless*, and the bodies of those deemed deficient, less than, and lacking by whites.

Ethicist Irene Oh offers additional insights by urging us to think about what Christians and Muslims share in their views of self-sacrificial or dutiful love as they connect specifically to motherhood. In both Christian and Muslim writings and traditions, "mothers tend to be objectified as symbols of willing and selfless devotion."[12] However, women's own voices are largely absent in the formation of these symbols. If women were to be authentically included in the discussion, caregiving would be explored in all of its complexities and varied circumstances and contribute a depth of ethical richness to Christian concepts of dutiful love and self-sacrifice.

Nitzia Chama puts another face on people who provide essential and life-giving care for family members. A young woman in her thirties, Chama immigrated to the United States from Veracruz, Mexico, to pursue her dream of becoming an actor. She began to care for her grandparents when she became aware of their developing medical problems. Her grandfather, Papá Albanito, was diagnosed with diabetes, early stage Parkinson's disease, and Alzheimer's. Mamá Chuyita, her grandmother, has high blood pressure and arthritis. You can imagine the debilitating nature of just one of these medical conditions, but together, there was no way for her grandparents to survive without assistance. When interviewed by National Public Radio (NPR) about her feelings concerning juggling her own full-time job and serving as a caregiver for her grandparents, Chama said she does not think of caregiving as "a burden. Although it may be a sacrifice . . . [she] considers it to be the right thing to do."[13]

Chama's caregiving is the right thing to do, but that does not negate the fact that social attitudes and public policies in the United States unfairly value and place the burden of care almost solely on her as an individual. Families with mixed immigration status are much more vulnerable because they have more difficulty accessing health care. Chama's story is also much more common than my own. One-fourth of caregivers in the United States today are millennials, and more than half identify as African American, Asian American, or Latinx.

Rosemary Radford Ruether, an internationally known Christian feminist theologian, shares Marshall's conclusions when reflecting on the sacrifices she and her family make for her son, David, and recognizes the social and economic injustices embedded in our health care system and the care industry. David is schizophrenic. With his input, Ruether wrote the book *Many Forms of Madness: A Family's Struggle with Mental Illness and the Mental Health System*, which is about her experience trying to understand schizophrenia and how she and her family worked together to attend to David's needs with limited help from a broken mental health system. David is extremely dependent on his family and lacks the capacity to organize himself. There was an era in David's life when he started doing flips. No one ever really understood why he started flipping. Sometimes he seemed to want to surprise a companion. At other times, he might go to the extreme of flipping off a second-story balcony inside a communal home. Ruether surmised that David wanted to return home.

As the parent of three children, she determined over time that she had to develop both "grace and limits" with David so that he would not "so absorb their energies that we would have no life of our own."[14] It is clear that she and her family make sacrifices to love and care for David, but at the same time, she insists on affirming his abilities, not just his need, and recognizes that dutiful love also incorporates mutuality.

Finding places for David to live where he can develop his own abilities, discover affirmation, and involve himself in community is an ever-present challenge. Cost is a factor. Some of the facilities Ruether describes tend to maintain the "status quo" and reinforce economic injustices by relying on social hierarchies, employing "mostly immigrants without any special job training to serve as caretakers."[15]

These narratives demonstrate some of the complexities in interpersonal care and underscore the larger social and economic context in which care-givers act. Nancy Fraser, a social theorist and feminist philosopher, says that we are in a crisis of care in contemporary Western late-stage capitalist societies. Fraser is a leading voice among social reproduction theorists. Social reproduction theory provides a lens through which we can better understand how social, economic, and political systems perpetuate inequalities based on race, ethnicity, age, national identity, gender, sex, physical and mental health, and class. Social, economic, and political constraints shape the strategic choices we all are forced to make regarding caregiving just as much as Christian norms for self-sacrificial and dutiful love. Capitalism only values labor that contributes to the means of production even though it relies on the unpaid labor of many people involved in life-sustaining and provisioning work as caregivers of children, people with mental and physical impairments, elderly family members, and others. Sustaining life requires the collaboration of a large network of people and a planet on which we must depend in order to maintain the conditions of existence.

Our current economy is driven by neoliberal economic policies that promote "state and corporate disinvestment from social welfare," placing more of the burden of caregiving on individuals and families.[16] Those with significant wealth and access to health insurance can pay or use benefits to employ caregivers outside of their family to assist them. Those without the financial means to pay for caregivers on their own or who cannot afford or lack access to health insurance are caught in the difficult space of working harder and harder to make ends meet and being forced to master multiple roles. Thus the growing wealth gap in the United States translates into a staggering care gap.

Worldwide, women form the bulk of providers of informal care for children, elderly family members, and people with mental and physical impairments. Sixty percent of all caregivers in the United States are women; 40 percent are men. Women in Organisation for Economic Co-operation and Development (OECD) countries spend an average of four and a half hours a day doing unpaid work, compared to slightly more than two hours a day for men. Additionally, women make up two-thirds of the health and social workforce.[17]

In the United States, women also dominate the long-term care industry and hold almost 90 percent of jobs in that sector, even though more men are entering into this segment of the workforce.[18] Elder care is one of the sectors of the economy that is expected to grow rapidly in the coming decades. The US Department of Labor projects that 1.6 million jobs will be added in fields related to elder care by 2024. The Institute for Women's Policy Research reports that the care workforce grew among all major racial ethnic groups, but the share of workers identifying as Latinx or multiracial grew by five to six times as much as those identifying as white.[19] Moreover, women in the care industry, even when they are well educated, live with higher rates of poverty than their male peers, and these jobs can have their own significant financial and health risks.

No matter where you live in the world, the current social, economic, and political environment will make it difficult to challenge stereotypes of and the stigma associated with mental illness and transform the contexts in which we conceptualize and practice dutiful love and caregiving. Scholars in disability studies observe that disability itself is a stereotype and trope used to mark elements in our society that are unwanted and to enforce a particular social order. Much of the conversation about caring for people with serious mental illness remains behind closed doors and hidden in the crawl spaces of different households because of the stigma associated with psychiatric disability. Disability studies and feminist, womanist, and postcolonial theories offer essential tools to interpret the context and humanize the conversation. Distinctive elements related to the lived reality of serious mental illness and the context of caregiving require careful examination and must be incorporated into our theological and ethical reflections on self-sacrifice, dutiful love, and caregiving. Therefore, narrating the embodied stories of individuals with serious mental illness and their family caregivers is an essential element in this book and to developing a concept of self-giving as an alternative way of living out dutiful love.

While writing this book, I interviewed more than twenty people from families affected by serious mental illness, mostly siblings who volunteered to be my conversation partners. When conducting these interviews, I wanted to find out more than whether others shared similar experiences with me. I wanted to deepen my own and our larger collective understanding of how mental illness affects an entire family system and the context in which members of a family care for each other. There are many elements to what psychologists and sociologists call the "family burden" of mental illness.

Our relationships with our siblings can be the longest we experience in our lives. However, in some ways, siblings are the least visible to others in the role they play as caregivers. Siblings must do much more than learn to cope in early life with a brother or sister's symptoms and their impact on the family. They may also need to take on caregiving responsibilities and learn to deal with a broken mental health system, experience their own trauma, and confront secondary stigma. Stories of siblings and other family members told in their own words provide a narrative thread woven throughout the chapters of this book. These stories lend witness to the chaos experienced within families affected by serious mental illness. They name both the fears and joys that siblings have when taking on caregiving responsibilities and highlight the larger context in which families make decisions about caregiving. Stories about the complicated lives of people with chronic physical and mental illness and the choices that caregivers are forced to make best show the places where the social fabric of care has unraveled for all of us.

The Vulnerability of Individuals with Mental Illness

On a social level, we are in the midst of a critical time to deal with questions about dutiful love, caregiving, and serious mental illness. People with serious mental illness all around the world are vulnerable; they are among the most economically and socially marginalized populations. Researchers Richard Wilkinson and Kate Pickett suggest that more than half of all US adults will suffer from a mental illness over their lifetimes.[20] Less than half of adults who experience mental illness get treatment in a given year. A larger percentage of white adults experiencing serious mental illness (50 percent) get treatment compared to those who identify as Asian American (23 percent), Black (33 percent), Latinx (34 percent), and LBGTQIA (49 percent).[21] According to research done by the Centers for Disease Control and Prevention (CDC), suicide rates have increased 30 percent between 2000 and 2016.[22] About 10 percent of children ages three to seventeen have "moderate or severe difficulties in 'the areas of emotions, concentration, behavior or being able to get along with others.'"[23] NAMI reports that in the United States, 20 percent of youth ages thirteen to eighteen live with a mental health condition. Suicide is the third-leading cause of death among youth ages ten to twenty-four; 90 percent of those young people who died by suicide had an underlying mental illness.[24] Youth and young adults between the ages of fifteen to twenty-four are "of particular concern, with increases in social media use, anxiety, depression, and self-inflicted injuries."[25]

A 2018 *Lancet* commission of twenty-eight medical experts conducted a study of global mental health and sustainable development worldwide and reported that every nation is a "developing country" when it comes to mental illness. The quality of care for people experiencing physical illness is routinely better than for those with mental impairments or emotional distress. Government policies and programs are "pitifully small." In some countries, "human rights violations and abuses persist . . . with large numbers of people locked away in mental institutions or prisons, or living on the streets, often without legal protection."[26]

Furthermore, Wilkinson and Pickett assert that countries with higher levels of income inequalities experience higher levels of mental illness. They argue, "Low position in the social status hierarchy is painful to most people, so it comes as no surprise to find out that the use of illegal drugs such as cocaine, marijuana, and heroin is more common in most unequal societies."[27] Social inequalities cultivate anxieties. For the last thirty years, income inequality has been growing in the United States by every statistical measure. *Fortune* reported in 2015 that the United States is the "richest, most unequal country" in the world.[28] Additionally, racism and homophobia are significant factors to consider. Negative stereotypes and the systemic exclusion of Black, brown, and LGBTQIA people create psychological distress and have measurable adverse consequences on these communities and our society as a whole. What will this mean for our future? For individuals affected by serious mental illness and their families, it means that the social fabric of care in the United States is nonexistent or full of holes, frayed, damaged, and desperately in need of thread for mending.

Discerning the Call of Christian Communities and Other Organizations in This Context

Communities of faith can be a real source of support for individuals affected by serious mental illness and their family members. Jesus announces the beginning of his public ministry in Matthew, Mark, and Luke by gathering disciples and proclaiming that he comes to release the captives, bring good news to people living in poverty, and heal every disease (Matthew 4:23–25; Mark 1:14–28; Luke 4:14–30). His announcement is a sort of mission statement for communities of faith.

No one can doubt the kind of precarious circumstances in which people with serious mental illness and their families live and the importance of the Christian call to bring good news and healing. In the last thirty years, local congregations, denominations, ecumenical and interfaith groups, and other religiously affiliated institutions have made significant and noteworthy efforts to collaborate and partner with mental health groups and social service organizations to advance a number of initiatives to address the circumstances of individuals with mental illness and their families. Examples include Pathways to Promise, NAMI FaithNet, and Mental Health Ministries. A great deal of recent research attests to the vital role that spirituality plays in the treatment of mental illness. *The Handbook of Religion and Mental Health* edited by Harold Koenig outlines and identifies trajectories in the explosion of research that began in the 1980s to explore the relationship between spirituality and mental health.[29] These efforts attest to the potential of communities of faith and other religiously affiliated organizations and institutions to be leaders in creating change. Communities, organizations, and institutions can cultivate a new and more just culture of caregiving and support. Religious belief contributes to one's sense of meaning and purpose, helps shape a positive worldview and provide hope, and is an important coping mechanism and resource for many people with serious mental illness and their families.

At the same time, much more work needs to be done to equip families to challenge the ways our society uses disability to stereotype and justify discrimination and to deal adequately with the wide variety of obstacles they are forced to confront. A sizeable amount of research lends witness to the persistence of the stigma associated with mental illness within congregations as well as other social institutions. Siblings of people affected by serious mental illness whom I interviewed consistently validated this research. They often expressed that they believed it was necessary to keep the mental illness of a family member a secret from their church and felt isolated within their community of faith. For example, Annie, a woman now in her fifties, first began to recognize her father's serious mental illness when she was in middle school and he made an unsuccessful attempt at suicide. Her father stayed on the church's prayer list for weeks. Her mother told her that if any members of the congregations asked about why her father needed prayer, she should tell them that he had an "allergic reaction" to medication. Annie said, "I kept it to myself."

Adelle Banks, a journalist for the *Religion News Service*, recently reported that "only one-fourth of congregations have a plan in place to assist families of the mentally ill."[30] That same study found that even the 66 percent of pastors who mention mental illness in sermons do so only "rarely." Pastor R. Abraham observes that religious leaders often do not receive the training and exposure they need to deal effectively with mental illness, which "may translate to careless attitudes towards people with mental illness in congregational settings."[31]

My effort, then, in this book is to adopt two main goals. First, I want to stimulate your reflection on the many ways that our theological traditions, rituals, and practices both disempower or disable and empower people with serious mental illness and their caregivers. Second, I aim to invite, excite, and empower you to venture into the stories and lives of individuals struggling with serious mental illness and to accompany them and their caregivers in their journey, to nurture belonging within communities in which you are involved, and to advocate for social change.

Chapter Outline

Many distinct and significant facets must be considered when developing a conversation about mental illness, its treatment in theology and within churches, and the contemporary circumstances and needs of individuals and family members who take on a caregiving role. I will develop this conversation in three parts to allow you as the reader to explore the interrelated but distinct facets of a complex and challenging problem.

Part 1, "Heading into Households and Crawl Spaces," turns your attention to the contemporary stigma and shame surrounding mental illness and introduces secondary stigmatization for family members. Chapter 1, "Being Parents and Children in a Culture of Stigma and Shame," focuses on the stories and experiences of individuals struggling with mental illness and their parents, lifts up studies of stigma beginning in the 1940s and 1950s, and discusses the urgent need to address stereotypes. The second chapter, "Siblings Naming Their Own Experiences," draws on interviews I conducted with siblings between June 2019 and August 2020. These siblings spoke about not feeling safe to "willingly share" their experiences for fear of how others would react, never "feeling community" from family or church, and being forced into the position of a passive observer as activity in the household unfolded. These experiences leave an indelible imprint on siblings' lives and the entire family system. Siblings also reflected in these interviews on how these relationships expanded their sense of self, expressions of spirituality, and understanding of God's providence and care.

Listening to the stories of other siblings and considering my own experiences led me to research and connect "History and Current Circumstances," the subject of part 2. Chapter 3, "A Brief Overview of the Treatment of People with Serious Mental Illness in the US Context," underscores pivotal figures and moments in the history of madness that continue to inform our current context of care. I pay special attention to the responses of Christian theologians and religious leaders to medical and scientific advances. In the West, Christianity and science are grounded in similar assumptions about human nature and ideas about order in the universe. As a result, advances in scientific and medical approaches to mental illness have not significantly altered the dominant view of what is "normal." Moreover, approaches to treating or caring for people with mental illness have remained hauntingly consistent over the course of time.

Through the early decades of the twentieth century, treatment focused on isolating people with mental illness in hope of restoring them to a "normal" state of health. The pursuit of curing mental illness moved beyond isolation to the use of psychotropic drugs and to the extremes of electric shock therapy, surgery, and compulsory sterilization by the mid-twentieth century. By the 1960s, *institutionalized care* became synonymous with *abuse*. Deinstitutionalization sought to empower people with mental illness, but communal homes and other programs never received adequate funding. As people were released from state hospitals, they did not always get enough financial and other kinds of support needed to prevent them from being forced onto the street or winding up in prison. Ultimately, the majority of Christian theologies, religious leaders, and faith communities embraced medical explanations and the scientific approach to mental illnesses without transforming the theological descriptions of the human that first created disability as a social construct.

A tremendous issue for individuals affected by serious mental illness and their families is the lack of social safety nets. Chapter 4, "Prescription for Poverty," highlights the systemic and structural causes of poverty among people with mental illness, the impact of neoliberalism on mental health policies in the United States, and how poverty and social inequalities contribute to mental illness. There are many reasons for such high rates of poverty among people with mental illness, including systemic and structural causes, social attitudes and the stigma associated with mental illness, able-bodied norms for work, and the ways in which poverty and wealth inequalities impact our overall physical and mental health.

The third part of this book emphasizes "Empowerment, Alternatives, and Advocacy." Chapter 5, "Biblical Threads of Empowerment," invites you to read biblical stories while keeping the perspectives of people with mental illness and siblings' descriptions of their own experiences at the forefront of your mind. I explore Greco-Roman concepts of ideal minds and bodies and how they shaped attitudes toward and treatment of people with disabling and disfiguring conditions in the ancient world. A biblical thread of empowerment is woven throughout the stories as God's character and concern are revealed by affirming the whole creation in God's image. God partners with the creation to bring meaning from the chaos of human experience and expand communities of care for people made vulnerable by social attitudes and beliefs. Jesus and Paul confront physiognomy, an ancient pseudoscience used to explain differences in human physical traits and determine how a person's appearance revealed their inner moral qualities.[32] In the biblical narrative, people with mental and physical impairments are agents of change and reveal the character of God and are not reduced to their "blemishes." "Communities of Empowerment and Belonging," the sixth chapter, picks up the empowerment thread. I offer several examples of communities throughout history that took an alternative approach to caregiving, such as Bethel, Geel, L'Arche, and Dismas Charities—the Diersen House. The good news for individuals and families shared in these two chapters is found in activities that calm the storms of chaos they experience in their lives, expand communities of care, and transform an ordering of households that privileges the bodies of some members over others. Chapter 7, "Cultivating Belonging and Practicing Intentional Prayer and Advocacy," invites you and your faith community, educational institutions, or other organizations in which you are involved to journey in solidarity with individuals and families affected by serious mental illness and take on a cause greatly in need of attention. In my reading of the Gospel stories, Jesus does more than act compassionately toward the demon possessed; he enters into their experiences, gets into the boat with them, and stills the storms of chaos surrounding them and their families. This final chapter incorporates Erik Carter's research on ten dimensions of belonging, examines these dimensions in light of the stories told by siblings of people with serious mental illness, and calls on communities of faith to enter into the work of weaving a social fabric of care and empowerment for individuals with serious mental illness and their families. Additional resources at the end of the book encourage individual and group reflection, offer a model for conducting an inventory of language and practices used in your congregation or organization, and provide a list of statements made by religious bodies that can be a resource for you.

———

Our most passionate human pursuits emerge from the questions that we find most difficult to answer. The silence and stigma surrounding serious mental illness in my family have become too great a burden to bear for me as a sibling. As a scholar of theology and Christian ethics, I am unable to accept the traditional theological explanations of disability and madness, concepts of self-sacrificial love, and the public policies that try to fit people with serious mental illness into boxes and checklists made for those with minds and bodies that are valued by society as ideal. Nonetheless, the church as a body of people gives me tremendous hope because on many occasions, it still brings me good news. I am hopeful because people in churches can model self-giving in life-restoring ways and weave together a fabric of caregiving as they interpret the meaning of Jesus's story.

When my daughter was born, our church celebrated her birth by bringing us gifts. One of the most treasured gifts was a peach blanket a friend named Carrie knitted while participating in a group that made beautiful handmade items as a symbol of ongoing love and support. When my husband's aunt and uncle became sick, the congregation we attended made prayer quilts large enough to warm them during the long days of recovery. Individual members of the congregation tie a knot in the strings sewn every few inches on a prayer quilt. Each knot represents a communal commitment to caregiving. I know many tailors, knitters, and weavers willing to take things apart when they become worn, out of style, or no longer useful. My mother helped me do this many times when I was first learning to sew. Sometimes fabric is reusable, and you can piece it together to create something altogether different. At other times, threadbare fabric needs to be thrown away. I invite you to join with me in pursuing the threadbare places in our Christian views of self-sacrificial love and charity for people affected by serious mental illness. My hope is to gather threads of self-giving, mutuality, reciprocity, and belonging so that a social fabric of empowerment can be woven by and wrapped around these individuals and their families.

PART I

Heading into Households and Crawl Spaces

CHAPTER ONE

Being Parents and Children in a Culture of Stigma and Shame

Stigma (etymology: Greek)

A mark made upon the skin by burning with a hot iron (rarely, by cutting or pricking), as a token of infamy or subjection; a brand. Also figurative.

Figurative. A mark of disgrace or infamy; a sign of severe censure or condemnation, regarded as impressed on a person or a thing; a "brand."

—*Oxford English Dictionary*

A lot of attention is given in our society and in Christian congregations to considering different types of families and ways of organizing family life and to ensuring for their well-being. Ethicist Gloria Albrecht makes the case that these debates about families in church and society often assume a particular form "as an ideal in contrast to which other forms of family have been found deficient, even dysfunctional."[1] "Ideal" families are not dependent on others to ensure their own well-being or provide for the needs of all members. "Good" parents produce children who are seemingly free from problems, prevent them from living in poverty, protect them from violence, and ensure their educational success. It is also quite common in our culture for successful children to be used as evidence of good parenting. Think about the many promotional posts made by parents on social media of children winning academic awards, athletic contests, or other competitions. Assumptions made about "ideal" or "good" families rarely, if ever, incorporate serious mental illness.

Consider briefly the experiences of two mothers. Liza Long first began sharing her feelings about her son's serious mental illness by blogging. In her memoir, *The Price of Silence*, she writes, "I wanted to have the perfect family. . . . I thought I could wish my child well, that if I prayed hard enough, God would make it all better."[2] Long admits that it is hard for parents to talk "about their children in part because they fall victim to self-stigmatization. They are more than willing to blame themselves, and society at large is happy to reinforce the message."[3]

Another mother named Ruth participated in the interviews I conducted. Ruth's daughter has been diagnosed with Tourette's syndrome. Her tics involve blurting out cusswords at unpredictable times, regardless of the social setting. Ruth admits, "All kinds of things come out of her mouth, and it makes me uncomfortable. When I found out that there was medication available to mask the tics, I wanted it because it could save some social embarrassment. It is more than that," she observes. The medications "actually allow her to manage interactions in the world in a more regular way." At the same time, Ruth expresses a sense of guilt about wanting her daughter to take the medication, but she is concerned about whether her daughter will be accepted in different social environments. The stigma and shame associated with mental illness and neurodevelopmental disorders and the social pressure to live up to expectations to be the "good" and "ideal" parent and family or high-achieving kid lead to the concealment of many of the real issues families face on a daily basis.

Scientific investigations of public attitudes toward mental illness began in the United States in the 1940s and 1950s as part of the mental health and deinstitutionalization movement. The intention of these early studies was to try to understand the stigma surrounding psychiatric disability and the significant burden placed on their families so that people with mental illness could return to their homes and communities with the support they needed when released from state hospitals. In 1950, Shirley Star, a senior study director at the National Opinion Research Center, conducted the first nationwide research regarding the public's perception of mental illness. Star and her team conducted 3,500 interviews that incorporated vignettes describing conditions such as anxiety, schizophrenia, alcoholism, juvenile character disorder, and compulsive phobia. The research findings revealed that the public had little understanding of the enormity of the problem and exposed the "view of human nature and of human conduct deeply engrained in Western civilization."[4]

In her 1955 summary of the findings, Star identified the stigma associated with mental illness: "Given this orientation, it also follows that mental illness is a very threatening fearful thing and not an idea to be entertained lightly about anyone. Emotionally, it represents to people loss of what they consider to be the distinctively human qualities of rationality and free will, and there is a kind of horror in dehumanization. As both our data and other studies make clear, mental illness is something that people want to keep as far from themselves as possible."[5] The majority of those interviewed by Star and her team looked to psychiatric and medical professionals for a cure and believed that people with serious mental illness were best treated in psychiatric hospitals.

Stigma is a term derived from a Greek word that refers to a mark made by a pointed instrument or brand. In the ancient world, stigmas were visible signs of social disgrace used to highlight something unusual or bad about a person, lapses in their moral character, or their social status. Psychologist Stephen Hinshaw observes that "the very creation of a social fabric within a community emanates in part from the boundaries that separate acceptable from unacceptable attributes, traits, and behaviors—in other words in-groups from outgroups."[6] The construct of disability and the stigma associated with mental illness emerge out of a larger fabric of social relationships that can connect or separate people with physical or cognitive impairments to or from those who are considered able-bodied and able-minded. Those relationships can function to privilege some at the expense of the exclusion and disadvantage of others.

Researchers have repeatedly shown since the early studies of the 1940s and 1950s that mental illness is "the most disturbing type of disability-related condition for the general public."[7] When a person is stigmatized by a disability, groups in positions of social power create boundaries to "exclude the 'infectiousness' of perceived stigma."[8] For example, *insane*, *moron, crazy, retard, feeble-minded*, and *lunatic* were once medical terms used to diagnose intellectual and developmental disabilities and serious mental illnesses. Today, we recognize how these words represent social attitudes toward people with mental impairments and intend to distance them from their "able-minded" peers. Another contemporary example of this is the symbol used to designate "handicap" parking, which creates a visible image that associates disability with limitations of physical mobility and the use of a wheelchair. Most of these types of labels and images urge us to reduce a person with disabilities to their "broken part."

Chapters 1 and 2 of this book explore the stigma associated with serious mental illness in the US context and share stories from the perspectives of individuals with serious mental illness and their parents and siblings. My intention in presenting these stories is to better understand the experience of stigma shared by these individuals and families and how boundaries that separate acceptable from unacceptable attributes, traits, and behaviors unravel the social fabric of care.

Most of the comments incorporated in these chapters were made by siblings growing up in families affected by serious mental illness whom I interviewed between June 2019 and August 2020. Their accounts represent the experiences of more than twenty families. You can find the questions asked during the interviews in the "Additional Resources" section at the end of this book. Some additional quotations are gleaned from parents who participated in the interviews because their children were under the age of eighteen and are taken from other sources, including journals and magazines, newspaper articles, blogs, and books.

The siblings whom I interviewed were all volunteers and responded to several invitations I made and posted on social media or after being encouraged to participate by friends or colleagues. Their identities are kept confidential here. All names have been changed to protect the identities of the participants and their family members. On occasion, I have changed the details of their stories in order to ensure confidentiality. The majority of siblings whom I interviewed identify as white. Fewer participants identify as Black or Asian. Most also identify as female. These siblings live primarily in the United States and represent northeastern, southeastern, midwestern, and western regions. They come from both urban and rural areas. A few of the interviewees are from Europe. The participants span three generations and range in age from eleven to over sixty.

In addition to including the testimonies of siblings, one thing that makes my exploration of these stories distinct when compared to studies done in psychology or the social sciences is that I also consider how Christian beliefs, doctrine, and practices play powerful roles in shaping our concepts of the "good" family, mental and physical health, and dutiful love and charity and informing stigma. Our religious identities are woven together with race, ethnicity, and social class as well as larger cultural values of individualism, independence, and self-control. I mentioned earlier that sharing stories of individuals and families affected by serious mental illness is a perilous venture because vulnerable people take on what may feel like an unreasonable risk. I also think it is important to observe that the way disability is presented by parents and siblings will often fail to challenge and push beyond the social constructions of normal and healthy as able-bodied and disabled as abnormal, even though the desire to do so is clear in their testimonies. I attribute this to the fact that most of the siblings whom I interviewed live in the present moment because of the immediacy of providing for basic needs. So their narratives will do more to highlight systemic failures, stigma, and stereotypes. However, unraveling the attitudes, concepts, beliefs, rituals, and practices that stigmatize and shame is essential to spinning the new threads needed to weave a social fabric of empowerment for people with serious mental illness and their families.

Labeling

The American Psychiatric Association (APA) published the first edition of the *Diagnostic and Statistical Manual of Mental Disorders* (DSM) in 1952, around the same time that the first nationwide studies of stigma were being conducted. Mental health professionals created the DSM after World War II largely because the Department of Veterans Affairs needed a common way to address the mental health issues that returning soldiers were facing. The manual relied on symptoms to develop a common language for diagnosing and naming behaviors considered aberrant as well as identifying intellectual disabilities. Prior to World War II and the DSM's publication, teaching centers across the United States designed their own systems and ways of naming mental illnesses, using terms such as *idiocy/insanity, mania, melancholia, monomania, paresis, dementia, dipsomania,* and *epilepsy.* Now in its fifth edition (DSM-5), the DSM is sometimes referred to as "the therapist's bible." Diagnoses are helpful in identifying approaches to treatment, especially when they enable individuals to gain control over their own circumstances. However, many raise questions about the harmful effects of labeling human characteristics as aberrant and deviant and the tendency to reduce a person's identity to a diagnosis. As a parent, Liza Long describes the DSM as "the equivalent of a crude hand ax trying to do a laser cutter's precision work."[9]

Labels become the means to mark and define difference and norm-defying behaviors but also connect to a particular understanding of ideal human nature and social power and views of right and wrong, healthy and sick. Developing a common way of naming various forms of mental disorders is not completely objective and colors the lens through which society views certain behaviors as nonnormative. This naming also plays a role in stigmatizing some of the natural tendencies and characteristics of people. The definitions can contribute to the disablement of people with serious mental illness because they move certain behaviors out of the "realm of cultural or moral standards and into the scientific domain of disease states."[10] When the DSM-5 was published, the British Psychology Society wrote to the APA with this complaint: "Clients and the general public are negatively affected by the continued and continuous medicalization of their natural and normal responses to their experiences."[11] In this case, the medicalization of serious mental illness can overstep its limits.

Scholars in the field of disability studies challenge us to think beyond medical and social-scientific concepts of and approaches to disability. Disability studies is part of a larger political movement that claims disability as a positive social value and affirms the right of people with disabilities to name their own identities and define their experiences. These scholars and activists assert that the concept of disability itself is a stereotype largely mediated by medicine, psychology, and pharmacology.[12] The medical model focuses a microscope on bodily "abnormalities." Douglas Baynton, Lennard Davis, Jay Timothy Dolmage, Margaret Price, Rosemarie Garland Thomson, and others challenge us to affirm people with disabilities as meaning makers and agents of change. The concept of disability often assumes that there is a common identity that people with physical and mental impairments share. However, stigma is the primary common ground shared by people with very diverse experiences of disability.

Stereotypes Reduce Complex Human Identities to a Disability

Pernicious stereotypes of people with various disabilities mark them as incompetent, weak, and perpetually childlike, even in adulthood, and reduce disability "to a mere state of impairment or . . . disqualifying defect, retributive punishment, threat, contagion, torment or senseless fate."[13] In addition, the majority of US Americans associate mental illness with violence. These stereotypes place a great deal of pressure on people with disabilities. They impact their interactions with key power groups such as teachers, landlords, employers, police, clergy, church members, and mental and physical health providers. Stereotyping can prevent them from fully participating and flourishing in their communities and achieving important life goals.

Moreover, studies show that race, ethnicity, gender, and social class compound the experience of disability. Researchers use the term *double burden* to describe being a member of a racial ethnic minority group and having a physical or mental impairment. Data made available after the passage of the Patient Protection and Affordable Care Act reveals that "members of racial and ethnic minority groups who have a disability face greater health disparities and inequalities than do their peers without a disability." People of color "with both mobility limitations and minority status experienced worsening health, more difficulty with activities of daily living, depressive symptoms, diabetes, stroke, visual impairment, obesity, low participation in physical activity, and low workforce participation."[14]

Being minoritized and devalued because of your race or ethnicity can also adversely affect your mental health.

One of the most powerful stories I have heard about stigma was told by a young woman who participated in the Valparaiso Project at St. Andrews Presbyterian College. The Valparaiso Project was a year-long study designed to provide students at the college with an opportunity to study Christian practices from the perspective of people with physical and learning disabilities. At the end of the study, the students who took part decided that they wanted to produce a video that incorporated interviews of other students with disabilities across the campus who also talked about their experiences in Christian communities of faith. Laura and Jennifer H. were twins who participated in the study. Both moved about with the assistance of motorized wheelchairs. At that time, Laura and Jennifer were about nineteen years old. Interviewers asked a series of questions about students' experiences, including one exploring "hurtful experiences in Christian communities." Jennifer said, "One of the most hurtful experiences I have ever had didn't even happen in a church." Like many teenagers, she and her sister enjoyed going to the mall to shop when they had some spare time. One afternoon, they were wheeling into a department store to do some shopping when someone who identified herself as a Christian stopped to talk with them. The woman asked if she could place her hands on their shoulders to pray for God to heal them. She was clueless about the offensive nature of her request and thought she was acting out of compassion. Not only did the woman ask for unreasonable access to their bodies, but she reduced Laura and Jennifer to objects and diminished the depth of their lives to a single narrative of suffering.

To Disclose or Not to Disclose?

People with mental illness and their families are deeply aware of stereotypes that inform discriminatory practices and policies. For example, people with serious mental illness frequently lack equal and fair access to housing and employment that pays a family-sustaining wage. They are often at an increased risk of homelessness and of being victimized by crimes. Courts in the many US states can declare people with mental illness "mentally incompetent," "insane," "idiotic," or of "unsound mind" and take away their right to vote.[15] Other rights may be curtailed or restricted, such as the right to a basic education, to obtain a driver's license, or to maintain custody of one's children. The hidden pressure to conceal one's disability becomes a protective and coping mechanism.

Consider the story of Reese and her family. Reese identifies herself as white, is about twelve years old, and has two siblings. She struggles with anxiety and depression. Her brother, Andrew, is the oldest sibling at fifteen, and Meara, her sister, is just nine years old. The family recently moved from Colorado to California because Mike, the father, was able to get a job with a higher salary and, most importantly, better health insurance and other benefits. Every member of the family described their home life as chaotic, including Reese. Amanda, the mother, is unable to work outside the home because of the unpredictability of Reese's behavior and the hostility that Reese experiences in different social environments.

Reese described what it is like to struggle with anxiety in this way: "Imagine all of your emotions all the time. Twenty-four-seven, you wake up just like sadness, happiness, anger—one day all the time. And it sucks a lot because you get really sad, and you think about all of these things that probably aren't true." Reese is reluctant to tell people how she feels. She said, "I definitely feel stigmatized—like I can't trust other people, especially when I am stressed." Her father, Mike, reflected on Reese's and the entire family's impulse to conceal the situation: "We have been very careful about who we let know. I don't think I have even told my parents [Reese's grandparents]. . . . I am not in a place to be able to deal with that right now. There is too much chaos in other ways."

Pushed to the Margins of the Classroom

Reese and her family reflected on her interactions with teachers and other school officials and felt that she was constantly misunderstood. People with serious mental illness may have some functional limitations that are stereotyped by teachers, staff, and other students and can affect their performance in the classroom in significant ways. As Reese put it, "[When I go into a panic attack,] my teachers will tell me we need to do this and this and this. Others go into problem-solving mode, and that doesn't help."

Neville, who is now in his fifties, also talked about what it was like to grow up with bipolar disorder and attention-deficit/hyperactivity disorder (ADHD) in the late 1960s and early 1970s: "I was born with it. So when I was younger, I didn't read terribly well at school and would skip over sentences. I guess it was the ADHD." Neville's first grade teacher required students to read aloud in front of the class. When Neville skipped over sentences, she would make him stop and go back. He continued to skip the sentences, and the teacher concluded that he was challenging her authority, so she punished him by making him stop reading with other students. Of course, the teacher's punishment made him stand out as different and pushed him to the margins of the classroom. Neville never felt like he could explain what was going on in his head to his teachers: "My brain has never worked in a linear pattern. I have always thought of my thoughts as tornadoes in my head. There is a logic there, but it is not a linear one." The teacher's decision affected his mastery of reading for years to come.

Many students struggle because of insufficient mental health resources, including counseling and psychiatric services. According to the Association for Children's Mental Health, "Only 40 percent of students with emotional, behavioral and mental health disorders graduate from high school, compared to the national average of 76 percent; and, over 50 percent of students with emotional and behavioral disabilities ages 14 and older, drop out of high school. This is the highest dropout rate of any disability group!"[16] The National Alliance on Mental Illness (NAMI) conducted a study of college students in 2011 and found that almost half of students with mental health issues don't ask for accommodations. More than a third of college students never inform their schools of issues with mental health. This can result in poor educational achievement.

High Unemployment and
Able-Bodied and Able-Minded Norms

Stigma also creates vocational limitations and makes it difficult for people with psychiatric disability to enter into the highly competitive primary labor market. Public health experts report that labor force participation for people with serious mental illness in the United States has "consistently hovered around 25 percent since the mid-1980s, and there has been a growing recognition that such pervasive unemployment is a significant problem."[17] Wyoming has the lowest rate of unemployment among people with serious mental illness at 56.1 percent. The states with the highest levels of unemployment among this group are Maine, 92.6 percent; West Virginia, 91.9 percent; Hawaii, 91.4 percent; Pennsylvania, 90.6 percent; and California, 90 percent. Among all people with serious mental illness, those with schizophrenia have the highest rates of unemployment.

Oftentimes, people with serious mental illness are held responsible for actions they cannot control, and these actions significantly influence employability decisions made by business managers and owners. For example, some people have diminished social inhibitions. This can make social interaction challenging and lead to misunderstandings. Those with schizophrenia may manifest the illness in different ways. Some experience paranoid delusions; others have disorganized thinking or extreme social anxiety. The stigma of the illness makes it difficult to disclose, especially because employers and employees often lack understanding. The unpredictability of the ways in which others will perceive and deal with mental illness can also be a major stressor.

Journalist Maria Hengeveld tells the story of Abdul-Ali Muhammad's struggle to hold down a job. Muhammad began hearing voices in 1975 after returning from a year in military service. For about ten years, he relied on alcohol and drugs to quiet his mind. He tried to quit but found that the voices just got louder. He made three attempts to commit suicide. Employment became one of the main keys to his recovery as he worked with the Veteran's Administration (VA) to get back on his feet. The VA helped him get housing and find a job that he could manage. He began working in a mailroom. After some success, the VA decided to move him into different positions. Muhammad ended up as a security guard, which required him to work on his own. One of his responsibilities was to monitor the grounds of a hospital at night. When he looked into the shadows, the sound of the voices in his mind increased. He became sick again. It was nearly impossible to explain to his supervisor why he could no longer serve in his position as a security guard. Neither Muhammad nor his boss could determine the most suitable job environment for him. Hengeveld reports, "Less than 2 percent of people with schizophrenia who are able and willing to work get the job support that they need to succeed."[18]

Challenging the Myth That People with Serious Mental Illness Are Just Lazy

Muhammad's story and Hengeveld's observation challenge us to debunk the myth that people drawing on Social Security Disability Income (SSDI) or with serious mental illness are lazy, unmotivated, or just don't want to work. While I am sure that one could find a few individuals who exploit the system, the vast majority of people with psychiatric disability are forced to live in the crawl spaces of the nation's economy. Good jobs that pay a living wage and provide for essential health care benefits and prescription insurance coverage are few and far between in the United States. Financial disincentives are also embedded in disability benefit policies, and the SSDI monthly income allocation itself is not enough to help anyone get out of poverty.

The lack of appropriate and effective support and rehabilitation for employment contributes significantly to high rates of unemployment, despite an awareness among mental health professionals that employment provides more than supplemental income. For centuries, theologians have honored the connection between work and the stewardship of one's God-given talents. A productive work environment is about much more than providing for one's material needs; it builds self-confidence, a support network, and a means for social inclusion. For nearly twenty years after the deinstitutionalization movement began, many communities had no programs to assist someone who had been released from a psychiatric hospital or was experiencing symptoms. The lack of work-related programs likely resulted in a consistent dismissal of the possibility for people with serious mental illness to work.

One study that interviewed people with serious mental illness indicated that "no one—neither psychiatrists, psychologists, social workers, case managers, nor family members—inquired about their employment histories or suggested that they begin to plan to earn a living in the future."[19] Neville (introduced previously) commented on feeling ashamed that he can't work: "I am not able to claim all of the knowledge I had when I got out of school, but that is just the way my brain ended up being." Employment is now understood to be central to enhancing the quality of life of people with disabilities. Various approaches are being developed, including individual placement and support, diversified placement, and transitional employment. However, studies show that very few people with serious mental illness are employed full time. It is estimated that about 22 percent are employed at any given time, with about half (12 percent) working full time.[20] Most of those jobs are in the secondary labor market—part time in entry-level, low-wage, minimum-benefit jobs with average annual earnings under $10,000.[21] Such minimal incomes do not provide the financial leverage needed to get ahead or live independently.

Stereotyped as Dangerous and Violent

Another obstacle people with serious mental illness face is the stereotype that they are dangerous and violent. This affects education, employment, access to good housing, and the realization of other important life goals. About 60 percent of US residents believe that schizophrenics are prone to violence, and around 32 percent associate major depression with violence.[22] In truth, the majority of people with serious mental illness are not violent. Statistics show that people with serious mental illness are a little less likely than others to be violent, but they are ten times more likely to be victims of violent crimes.[23] Only a small subgroup has violent tendencies, and a link has been made between violent tendencies and substance abuse. The MacArthur Violence Risk Assessment Study discovered that "31% of people who had both a substance abuse disorder and a psychiatric disorder (a 'dual diagnosis') committed at least one act of violence in a year, compared with 18% of people with a psychiatric disorder alone." Therefore, researchers conclude, "substance abuse is a key contributor to violent behavior."[24]

Neville lamented being stereotyped as dangerous and violent: "The one thing, stigma-wise, is that people are afraid of manic depressives. They always blame manic depressives for shooting up schools and stuff, but I am not violent. You have to have something else wrong with you." He tries to protect himself from these attitudes with nondisclosure: "I generally don't tell people because they are not that interested. Sometimes when I do tell people that I am bipolar, they admit they share the experience. But most express a lot of fear. You can see it on their faces."

The media plays a significant role in shaping public perceptions regarding the connection between serious mental illness and violence. Think about popular movies such as *One Flew over the Cuckoo's Nest*, *Psycho*, and *Fatal Attraction*. Who could forget the gripping scene of Glenn Close standing in the kitchen of her lover, scrapping a butcher knife against her thigh as blood drips down her leg? More recently, stories about school and other mass shootings often associate violence with untreated mental illness. Only about 14 percent of news stories offer reports about the successful treatment of mental illness, whereas around 55 percent discuss it within the context of a violent act.[25] However, researchers such as Michael Stone, professor of clinical psychiatry at Columbia University, have concluded that attention given to mass murders perpetrated by mentally ill people "has led to unwarranted stigmatization of the mentally ill as an inherently dangerous element in society."[26] A much more common trait among mass killers is that they are almost exclusively men who have a "history of hating women, assaulting wives, girlfriends, and female family members, or sharing misogynistic views online."[27]

Increased Urgency to Address Stereotypes

Camille Gear Rich and Elyn R. Saks, faculty of the University of Southern California School of Law, express a sense of urgency to address stereotyping people with serious mental illness as threats because it "grows even more deadly when combined with stereotypes about race and class."[28] For example, people who are homeless and mentally ill in the United States, a population that is disproportionately Black and male, come into frequent contact with the police. A 2015 study of fatal police shootings in Los Angeles reported that 33 percent involved people with some sort of serious mental illness. The *Washington Post* conducted a study of the fatal shootings by police officers during that same year and found that one-fourth of the individuals who were shot to death had serious mental health conditions. More recently, research by groups such as the Treatment Advocacy Center suggests that as many as half of all fatal police shootings involve people with untreated mental health conditions.[29] The Bureau of Justice Statistics reports that people incarcerated in state and federal prisons are nearly three times as likely to have a disability such as Down syndrome, autism, dementia, intellectual disabilities, and learning disorders; one in five has serious mental illness.[30]

Internalizing Stigma

The stigma associated with serious mental illness is so pervasive that people often internalize the stereotypes and perceptions held by others. This leads to low self-esteem and the failure to pursue work or to be included in different social groups, resulting in long-term negative consequences such as feelings of isolation, hopelessness, and despair. Kathleen Gallo wrote poignantly about how she internalized the stigma: "I perceived myself, quite accurately, unfortunately as having a serious mental illness and therefore as having been relegated to what I called 'the social garbage heap.' . . . I tortured myself with the persistent and repetitive thought that people I would encounter, even total strangers, did not like me and wished that mentally ill people like me did not exist. Thus, I would do things such as standing away from others at bus stops and hiding and cringing in the far corners of subway cars. Thinking of myself as garbage."[31]

Another dynamic to explore is the connection among racism, homophobia, and mental health issues. Stigma, discrimination, and systemic oppression create psychological distress. As a result, marginalized people experience double or triple oppression. Adult Black and brown people in the United States are 20 percent more likely to report serious psychological distress than adult whites. Nearly 40 percent of Black and brown people who also identify as LGBTQIA individuals will report experiencing psychological distress in a given year.[32]

The psychiatrist and political philosopher Frantz Fanon was raised in Martinique under French colonial rule. He articulated what is now considered a classic framework for understanding the relationship between systemic oppression and internalized oppression and how neuroses can be socially generated. When a group of people is devalued socially because of their race or ethnicity, and social, economic, and political institutions are created to privilege and maintain the superiority of a dominant group, those who are forced into a subordinate position are likely to internalize their own oppression and wrestle with mental health issues. For example, the internalization of whiteness as the ideal skin color can lead to efforts "to become as white as possible in order for social mobility or acceptance."[33] Today, a large proportion of non-European women resort to skin whiteners, which also negatively impact their physical health.

Among people with serious mental illness, the internalization of stigma and oppression can lead to self-violence. The greatest risk is for children and young adults. Hinshaw reports that "more than 30,000 [US] Americans commit suicide every year—with most of those related to serious mental disorder—almost double the number who die in homicides."[34] Suicide is the second leading cause of death among people ages twenty-five to thirty-four. One in three people diagnosed with schizophrenia will attempt suicide. Teenagers of color are about one and a half times more likely to attempt suicide than their white peers. In addition, people who identify as LGBTQIA are three times more likely to experience a mental health condition and four times more likely to attempt suicide than their peers who are straight.

Unintentionally Reinforcing Stereotypes and One Way to Challenge Them

Stereotypes of people with serious mental illness are sometimes unintentionally reinforced by religious communities. Consider, for example, one of the miracle stories often cited in study groups and sermons as an example of biblical teachings concerning the experience of people living with serious mental illness. The story of the Gerasene demoniac found in Mark 5:1–20 (see also Luke 8:26–37) is about a man afflicted by "unclean spirits" and "demons" who was forced by the community to live in the tombs among the ghosts. When the man sees Jesus and others approaching, he appears to lack all self-control as he shouts and swears, saying, "What have you to do with me, Jesus, Son of the Most High God? Swear to God that you won't torture me!" (Mark 5:7). This man "had been secured many times with leg irons and chains, but he broke the chains and smashed the leg irons. No one was tough enough to control him. Night and day in the tombs and the hills, he would howl and cut himself with stones" (5:4–5). Jesus frees the man from the unclean spirits by sending them a herd of pigs feeding on the hillside. The pigs rush down the hill and into the lake. When this event is reported to people in the surrounding town and countryside, they see the man "fully dressed and completely sane" (5:15), appear to be afraid, and ask Jesus to leave the region. Jesus gets into a boat and sends the man away to tell others what "the Lord has done for you" (5:19).

Challenging stereotypes and considering the impact of the interpretation of biblical stories like the Gerasene demoniac are essential to confronting the stigma associated with serious mental illness and empowering individuals and families. Ched Myers, for example, reads the story as a "politically evocative and symbolic critique of Roman occupation."[35] The Gerasene demoniac exhibits all the signs of "internalized oppression" resulting from the state of captivity in which the Romans force him to live. Christine Guth, a program associate for the Anabaptist Disabilities Network, offers another interpretation and hopeful response as she rewrites the story from the perspective of the man living in the tombs and emphasizes the trauma that living with a mental illness can cause. Guth imagines the many details Mark didn't share. The man describes what it feels like to be tormented by spirits and then to hear them depart like a thundering herd. Jesus sits with him for quite a while to talk about how long the spirits had been tormenting him. For the man living in the tombs, proclaiming "the truth—the whole truth—is essential."[36] He admits that while "Jesus drove the Legion out," he will likely "never be finished wrestling with the spirits that want to take Legion's place."[37] Guth's interpretation challenges many of the stereotypes described in this chapter and can be empowering as individuals, families, and other caregivers confront the reality that healing in the case of serious mental illness is a process, not an event, that "often involves one step backward for every two steps forward."[38]

Family Burden and Secondary Stigma

The social context and construct of disability extends beyond the experience of an individual to caregivers who are expected by the larger community to take on what sociologists and psychologists call family burden.[39] Since the mid-1950s and 1960s, family burden has been the subject of much study as researchers began to recognize the challenges and difficulties that families face because of attitudes toward those with serious mental illness and lack of social safety nets. Family burden refers to the impact of mental illness on work, income, children, relationships, and the overall health of family systems. Caregivers for people with serious mental illness experience a great deal of stress, both emotionally and financially. The disproportionate time investment required to meet the needs of one family member can make it difficult to build relationships with others. Parents and siblings fear social exclusion, feel emotionally isolated, and often try to conceal the serious mental illness from others in order to protect themselves—even though, I suggest, keeping these experiences under wraps seldom, if ever, helps. Siblings often harbor feelings of neglect. These forms of secondary stigmatization or secondary disability leave an indelible imprint on families.

Earlier, I reflected on the many different forms of love articulated and explored by philosophers and theologians. Dutiful or self-sacrificial love is most often referenced in relation to family life in Christian writings, although how this love is described may vary somewhat depending on the denominational tradition. Protestant theologians in the early twentieth century looked to family and other communal institutions for social regeneration. Social gospel theologian Walter Rauschenbusch wrote, "The home is the source of most of our happiness and goodness, and in the home we live communistically.... The income of the members is more or less turned into a common fund.... The housewife is the manager of a successful communistic colony and it is perhaps not accidental that our women, who move thus within a fraternal organization, are the chief stays of Christianity."[40] This patriarchal and overly romantic description of family responsibility and the duty to care for others endures in white, middle-class, Christian households. Furthermore, most theologians, religious leaders, and Christian communities fail to pay adequate attention to the gendered expectations of family responsibility and the larger context of social, economic, and political power relations in which caregivers act.

Parents and Partners

Growing up in a religious household, my faith tradition played a significant role in shaping my views of what a "good" family ought to look like. I don't remember a single explicit lesson on the "good" Christian family, but a lot of expectations were communicated in more subtle and indirect ways. Sermons preached, devotionals read, stories told in Sunday school settings, and activities in youth group encouraged me to think about the holy family, Mary, Joseph and Jesus; Timothy and his mother and grandmother; and Ruth, Naomi, and Boaz as models for family life. The predominantly white, middle-class, Southern Baptist churches I grew up in were more liberal than most, but the traditional nuclear white Protestant family was still the only model of domestic life that I remember being presented publicly. There were even more unspoken expectations for the families of ordained ministers and "PKs" (preachers' kids). Other

stories about siblings in the biblical narrative, such as the prodigal sons
and Mary and Martha, contributed to my family's idea of how siblings
ought to treat each other. Martha was the dutiful sister of Lazarus and
Mary of Bethany who welcomed Jesus into her home but occupied herself
with preparations for her guest and resented her sister for not doing more
to help. My mother's name was Martha, and honestly, she had much in
common with Martha of Bethany.

Dutiful love set the expectation for my mother's role in the family
from her childhood on. She celebrated that role some while resenting it
greatly. She was the oldest of three siblings who grew up in a working-
class family. Her younger sister, Charlotte, was sick most of the time
they were children, and my mother was often called on to help with
caregiving responsibilities. Charlotte also got a lot of things she wanted
because her parents wanted to make her feel better, whereas my mother
had to make her own way in life—find a job or do without. My mother's
father, whom I never met, was an alcoholic and commanded a lot of
household attention. When her parents divorced, my mother was always
the one expected to help whoever seemed to have the greatest need. She
resented that expectation most of her life. The resentment wasn't caused
by a lack of love. She didn't love her family any less than other people
do. The burden of family caregiving she shouldered meant that she had
to sacrifice other things she wanted for herself—going away to college,
earning a four-year bachelor's degree, and having her own career. She
never questioned that it was her duty to care for my brother throughout
his struggle with serious mental illness. My mother loved him greatly, but
at the same time, she needed life-restoring love to balance her sacrifices.
Research shows that the stigma felt by those caring for relatives with
mental impairments, particularly as parents, is "equivalent to the burden
of having a homeless relative and stronger than that associated with
having a relative with multiple sclerosis."[41] In 1999, NAMI conducted a
nationwide survey of 756 families affected by severe mental illness. The
study revealed that 70 percent of the parents experienced "severe marital
stress."[42] Fifty percent reported that they worried about aggression from
their child. Moreover, 37 percent of parents related that mental health
professionals had little to offer by way of help. Some studies suggest

that feelings of stigma and shame are intensified in families with higher levels of education.

Paying for and planning for lifelong care for people with physical disabilities, cognitive impairments, and serious mental illness is an immense task due to the lack of adequate mental health care, ever-decreasing social safety nets, and the limited availability of flexible work environments for caregivers. The systemic and structural causes of poverty among people with serious mental illness will be examined more in depth in chapter 4, but it must be noted here that a tremendous financial burden is placed on parents with a child who has a chronic health condition of any sort. The 1999 NAMI study also found that one in five parents "were forced to give up their children because they couldn't afford to pay for much-needed treatments and services."[43] In addition, one partner had to quit or take another job in 55 percent of families so that the child would get the support needed.

These conditions make it necessary for some parents to debate having a second child to ensure that someone is available for lifelong caregiving because of the lack of social safety nets for people with disabilities. Moreover, some parents consider having a third child so the "well" sibling is not left alone to shoulder the burden of care for the sibling with challenges.

Empowering individuals with serious mental illness and their families requires us to carefully interrogate the tropes and stereotypes of disability and to imagine a life together beyond roles into which we are compartmentalized. Considering the experiences of siblings is an essential aspect of this process of reexamination. The voices and experiences of siblings are largely neglected in studies of individuals affected by serious mental illness and their families, even though sibling relationships are some of the longest in our lives, and siblings are often expected to take on responsibilities as caregivers. In this role, siblings also remain largely invisible to counseling professionals, the medical community, and government agencies. The next chapter incorporates the stories of siblings as they name and describe their own experiences of secondary stigmatization as well as how their relationships with their brother or sister expanded their own sense of self and deepened their understanding of God.

CHAPTER TWO

Siblings Naming Their Own Experiences

My story will never be inseparable from my brother or from God. None of us are truly inseparable from each other and God—we belong to each other as one body.

—Grace

E arly studies attended to the impact of secondary stigma on parents and partners, but examining the experience of siblings is a relatively new area of research. Peter Burke, a professor of social work at Hull University in the United Kingdom, focuses his research on the entire family system, primarily caregivers for people with physical disabilities. Nevertheless, Burke's conclusions are just as relevant for families impacted by serious mental illness. Burke found that "approximately 80 percent of children with disabilities have non-disabled siblings."[1] He also discovered that a large majority of parents (about 80 percent) relied on their children without disabilities to help with caregiving responsibilities, which means that siblings' lives and relationships can be restricted.

In recent years, more attention has been given to serious mental illness and its impact on siblings who are not consistently struggling with their own mental health issues. These studies compare the lives of adults who had siblings with serious mental illness to those who did not. Having a sibling with a mental illness "can be a very difficult and traumatic experience that can negatively affect [one's] own health and well-being, the inter-sibling relationship and other family relationships."[2] Jaclyn Leith, Thomas Jewell, and Catherine Stein are clinical community psychologists who undertook a cross-sectional study of 242 siblings whom they refer to in the study as "well" siblings. Their intention was to learn more about these well siblings' attitudes toward their caregiving responsibilities as their parents aged. The study found that "poor sibling relationship quality during childhood and adolescence and differential treatment by parents can decrease well siblings' willingness to engage in caregiving in adulthood despite sociocultural or family expectations."[3] At the same time, siblings who are called on as caregivers feel a sense of guilt when they prioritize their own needs. In Leith, Jewell, and Stein's study, only about 21 percent of siblings take on the responsibility of becoming primary caregivers. Those who do are more likely to be people of color and women.

The stories that follow share some of the feelings and theological reflections expressed by siblings of people with psychiatric disability as they contemplated their own experiences. Sibling perspectives complicate this conversation and make it much more difficult to divide and categorize members of a family in terms of able-minded and well, mentally ill and sick. Nearly all of these siblings attest to the reality of secondary stigma. Several reflect on the tension they feel as they confront the social stigma associated with serious mental illness while at the same time loving their sibling as the unique person they are. Three siblings—Dorothy, Deborah, and Grace—express how their sibling relationship expands their own sense of self and idea of God's providence. Some also reflect on the importance of supportive and nurturing communities of faith and friends that help them challenge stereotypes of disability, confront the stigma, and empower them as caregivers by sharing in that duty. I make every effort in this chapter to present these experiences as they were shared with me by siblings whom I interviewed and change as few details as possible in order to maintain anonymity.

"My Sister Gets Anxiety Sometimes, and It Puts Some Stress on Me."

When caregiving responsibilities take a great deal of time due to limited support or because a family member demands a great deal of attention, it is quite common for siblings not experiencing the same issues to feel neglected or socially isolated as a result of competing interests within the family. Aiden is now eleven and his brother, Jordan, who has physical and intellectual disabilities, is eight. Aiden realizes that his brother has special needs and that Jordan "is treated differently than a regular kid because he needs more attention." Aiden loves his brother but also said, "It makes me feel sort of sad because I want to be involved in more stuff." Their mom, Julie, worries about Aiden getting "the short end of the stick." There are times that "he doesn't get to experience what other people do. Like when we have to cancel because his brother is sick. I remember one Friday, [Jordan] was sick, and [Aiden] said, 'I guess that means that we are stuck at home.'"

Neglect can also take a significant toll on siblings emotionally and physically. Andrew, who is now fifteen, described his sister Reese's behavior in this way:

> Before my sister started taking medicine, it would be really hectic and crazy all the time. My sister has anxiety. It is always really crazy after school. It kind of looks like her breaking down just out of nowhere. She would start crying a lot and get extremely sad easily even if I was trying to make a joke. Then she went to the mental hospital for almost a week. It was two weeks. We could all tell that no one was really happy with her going to the mental hospital even though we thought that was the real choice. Everyone got really angry with each other when she started going to the mental hospital. . . . It was a life-changing moment, a game changer for us, because it meant that there were some things that we couldn't talk to her about, and there were some things that we couldn't do anymore as a family.

Meara, the youngest sibling in the family, feels like her sister's anxiety puts some stress on her: "It is as if I feel like I should do something about it, but I don't know how. I get a little anxiety."

"I Absolutely Experienced [Secondary Stigma]."

Dorothy is a caregiver for her younger brother Peter, who was diagnosed as a teenager with schizoaffective disorder bipolar type. When I asked Dorothy if she experienced secondary stigma, she responded quickly to my question: "I absolutely experienced it. I have a pretty clear memory of it." The impact of serious mental illness was felt across the lines of different generations in Dorothy's family: "At fifteen years old, my mom explained to me that my dad had schizophrenia." He had been hospitalized when Dorothy was five, ten, and fifteen years old. She said, "I told one friend that my dad had schizophrenia, and she said, 'You mean like a psycho-killer in the movies?'" Dorothy realized almost immediately that it was best not to tell anyone else.

"The Constant Chaos and Piles of Clutter Made Me Never Want to Bring Anyone Home."

Life at home within families affected by serious mental illness can be unpredictable and chaotic. Nearly all of the siblings whom I interviewed talked about what it felt like to grow up in that environment, and many were afraid to bring friends home. Adair describes herself as a child of the 1950s. She grew up in a blue-collar household. Her father was a veteran who fought in Normandy in World War II. He was also known for spending evenings at the local bar. Adair explained, "I'm not excusing his alcoholism, but to think about what he must have gone through sort of makes you understand the need to self-medicate. But the mindset of my blue-collar family was 'You be a man' and 'Accept that as your lot in life.' If someone suggested that this man go to treatment, it would have absolutely crushed him. It was all about his manhood."

These ideas about masculinity and accepting one's lot in life shaped not only the way Adair's family responded to her father's alcoholism but also the way they dealt with the onset of her brother's mental illness. "My real introduction to mental illness was probably around twelve," Adair remembered. "I always knew some things weren't quite right, but at that time, I couldn't identify them using the language of mental illness." She first truly became aware of the mental illness that affected her family when she was an adolescent and started visiting friends in their households. She reported, "I recognized pretty quickly that their lives weren't as crazy as mine."

Another sibling, Eleanor, is now in her forties and being called on to serve as a caregiver for her older sister, Christina, in the wake of their parents' death. Christina is three years older than Eleanor and was diagnosed with bipolar disorder when they were in their late teens. However, symptoms began to appear much earlier. Eleanor described life in their childhood home as "chaotic and unpredictable." She said, "I always felt like I had to walk on eggshells." Christina had a tendency to talk a lot and spit out criticisms with the speed and intensity of an assault weapon. "You never knew when you were going to be the target," Eleanor remembered. Christina's mood swings and bouts with what the family called "sadness" at the time made it challenging for her to make friends.

As you might expect, Christina's erratic behavior consumed their parent's attention, leaving them little energy to deal with Eleanor's needs. Eleanor coped with and responded to what she simply called "the family situation" by becoming more independent and seeking opportunities to get out of the house. She said, "At that time, I didn't realize how sick [Christina] was, and so I just began to avoid her. I just needed to go on with my life. I didn't go home very often." Ultimately, Eleanor's coping mechanisms created a gulf between herself and her family.

"I Knew I Could Not Tell a Soul."

In my interviews, the stigma associated with suicide weighed heavily on siblings' decisions about whether to talk openly about the impact of mental illness on their families. Dorothy is now in her late forties and was already in college when her brother Peter experienced the onset of his mental illness. He made his first suicide attempt at the age of fourteen. Dorothy remembered what it was like to hear the news while she was away at school: "I was super involved in campus ministry at a premier Catholic university. I was staff for campus housing at my college, and my brother tried to commit suicide. I knew I could not tell a soul."

Adair's mother was eighty-two when her brother died by suicide. She described her mother as a "very devout Catholic—stoic and strong." Parish churches were in the midst of consolidation while her father and brother were dealing with mental health issues, and there were ongoing conversations about sex abuse scandals in the church. Adair's mother felt that she should keep some of her own emotions to herself so as to not add further stress within their congregation. Adair recalled, "My mother began to deteriorate rapidly after my brother's suicide. It was necessary then for me to step into the role of caring for her. . . . I don't think I ever got to grieve. Busyness took over. Responsibilities for family, a sick mother, completing a master's degree—it became really easy to sweep this whole thing under the rug."

Annie shared similar experiences as she discussed growing up in a household in which both her father and sister were diagnosed with bipolar disorder. Her father tried to commit suicide when she was in middle school. She first learned about his attempt from her uncle when he picked her up from school at the end of that day. Her uncle simply told her that her father "had an accident." Her mother later shared that "he overdosed." Annie's father languished for a few days in the hospital as he battled his self-induced coma. She remembered, "When they released him [from the hospital], there was no family counseling. Not even for my mom. They discharged him with some medications and that was it."

Annie and her family were members of a Lutheran church at the time. She said, "My dad was put in the church bulletin. He was on the prayer list. But because of the stigma around suicide, my mother told us just to tell everyone that he had an allergic reaction. So I kept it to myself." When Annie was in high school, her father made a second attempt and ended up not being able to work. Her parents divorced, and the family was forced to access public assistance, including food stamps. In the meantime, her sister was "diagnosed with depression."

Historically, the failure of Christian communities to grapple with the lived reality of mental illness has been enshrined in doctrinal teachings concerning suicide. The stigma associated with mental illness and suicide leads many people of faith to conceal mental health issues. The Roman Catholic Church, for example, once taught that suicide was a mortal sin because it was understood to be an act of the individual's will against God and therefore a violation of the fifth commandment. Thus funeral and burial services for someone who died by suicide could be withheld from the family.

Church leadership also felt the impulse to conceal mental illness. Mark Meade, assistant director of the Merton Center at Bellarmine University, explores the monastic censorship of the writings of Thomas Merton due to objections on moral or theological grounds. Meade has found that some of the material cut from Merton's published writings includes references to his many bouts with depression and to suicide ideation.[4] This form of censorship communicates more than moral or theological disagreement; it emphasizes that people called into religious vocations cannot be exemplary spiritual guides while at the same time struggling with depression, anxiety, or other mental health issues. Today, Roman Catholic teachings regarding suicide have changed, but the stigma remains. Protestants do not share the same concept of mortal sin but have not dealt with suicide any more effectively.

"What I Really Needed Was a God Able to Do Triage Every Day."

Later, Adair began to ask deeper theological questions about the serious mental illness affecting her family: "What kind of God would cause this to happen to a family? To a man who was a good man and tried his best to make his connection with a Catholic church but didn't have success? He was in and out of treatment his whole life. He so wanted to feel God's presence throughout his life but ended up losing his battle when he hung himself in the county jail."

Hans Reinders, a professor of ethics at the Free University of Amsterdam, gives some insight into why it is difficult for siblings and parents to grapple with the relationship between God and mental illness. Reinders observes that stories told by parents when they first learn about their child's physical, intellectual, or emotional disabilities usually start with an expression of devastation—"the feeling that the world is falling apart."[5] Parents ask, "Why me? Why my child?" One sibling named Ellen with whom I spoke had a similar reaction when her brother was born with an intellectual disability. She was about seven years old when she learned about his disability. The first questions she asked her mother were "What did I do wrong?" and "Is there something I can do to fix him?"

One of the reasons many Christians in Western society raise questions in this way is that we are conditioned to make sense of disability by trying to understand the meaning or purpose of it. Reinders suggests that these questions rest on the theological assumption that God intends for all bodies and minds to be free from impairments or disabling conditions. Therefore, when people and their bodies and minds don't fit dominant views of what society establishes as normal, their experiences are cast primarily as misfortune or suffering and can be linked theologically to a sense of divine punishment. Christianity, in this sense, has "a bad reputation" for addressing these questions.

Adair remembered, "All I ever got to talk about at church was blame and shame. I didn't need to talk about that; I felt plenty of that on my own. There wasn't a day that the church doors were open that my mother wasn't there." As the oldest daughter in the family, Adair thought her role "was to keep the family whole and holy. What I really needed was a God able to do triage every day."

"The Way I Functioned Was to Be a Fixer and a People Pleaser."

As you can imagine, no one could emerge from these experiences unscathed. Annie reflected, "It was all so draining. I was always the one who had to take care of everybody. That didn't fare very well for me. The way I functioned was to be a fixer and a people pleaser. There are a lot of long-term ramifications." Annie ended up leaving home to go to college at the age of eighteen and never turned back. However, these experiences left an indelible imprint on her and permeated relationships throughout her life even when she had her own family.

"You Have All These Thoughts about How Things Should Be. . . . And They're Just Not Going to Be."

The story of two more sisters and the complexity of their relationship captured the attention of *Kaiser Health News*. Jean and Ruby live in Clinton, North Carolina. Ruby has schizophrenia. However, things weren't always that way. Jean and Ruby were inseparable when they were children. It wasn't until Ruby was seventeen that she experienced depression after having her first child. Things in her life then took an unexpected turn. She later experienced a psychotic episode and was diagnosed with paranoid schizophrenia, which began a thirty-five-year downward spiral. After years of inconsistent treatment, Ruby couldn't manage her medications or self-care, lost custody of her child, and ended up homeless on the streets. Jean built a successful career during that time and ended up working in mental health after watching her sister's decline and years of struggle. Jean traveled from her home in Maryland so that she could scour the streets in search of her sister. She finally found her and then fought to become Ruby's legal guardian. Ruby now resides in an assisted living facility. Jean said, "You have all these thoughts about how things should be, could be, how you'd like them to be. And they're just not going to be."[6]

"[I Was] Torn about How Much I Should Personally Sacrifice."

The people with whom I spoke had conflicted feelings about taking on caregiving responsibilities. Several did not see caregiving as a real choice because of the fear of what might happen to their sibling—poverty, homelessness, jail time. One participant of the Leith, Jewell, and Stein study clearly stated, "I feel torn about how much I should personally sacrifice when it comes to meeting the needs of my ill sibling."[7] This sister's observation lends support to my claim that concepts of self-sacrificial and dutiful love fail to capture the reality of people's lived experiences. Social, economic, and political power relations also shape our expectations of family roles and responsibilities. Often, they are gendered expectations through which women are asked far more frequently to sacrifice themselves out of the duty to care for others. These sacrifices can come at a cost. Siblings who do act as adult caregivers tend to complete fewer years of education, are twice as likely to be unemployed, and experience greater psychological distress. In addition, taking on caregiving responsibilities can create more conflict within families for a variety of reasons, particularly with parents.

"I Think the Hardest Part about This Has Been My Mom. . . . She Has Been More in the Way."

Glenn is now in his early sixties and recognizes that his mother is aging. He and his sister are feeling the weight of the expected burden of care for their brother, who has paranoid schizophrenia and has lived with their mother for decades. There are many tasks awaiting Glenn and his sister, including convincing their mother she can no longer be the primary caregiver, seeking power of attorney, finding a group home, moving their brother, and seeking broader networks of support. Of course, all of these tasks must be done with the hope that their brother will "stick to the plan." Glenn said, "I think that the hardest part about this has been that my mom has been at the center of it. I think she has been more in the way than she has actually helped. My sister and I are going to try to work on a plan." In the area where his mother and brother live, there are few options for communal care, and she has difficulty handing over what she sees as her responsibility for their brother. What Glenn named at the end of our conversation was an intense loneliness. "Even as a family, there is a profound loneliness about this," he said. "You don't actually know what to do."

"Who Would Want to Marry Me Knowing This Will Become Their Problem down the Line?"

Harriet expressed her fears about taking on the responsibility for her older sister when her parents die. Her sister has lived with her parents for decades. She has anxiety, bipolar disorder, and learning disabilities. She can't drive, can't work, and can't remember to take her many medications. "I love her," Harriet said. "But recently, I've been having really dark, negative thoughts about what will happen to me when my parents are no longer with us. I'm frankly terrified. . . . Who would want to marry me knowing this will become their problem down the line?"

"You May Not Want to Have Kids with Me Because of My Family History."

Similar questions entered Dorothy's mind when she was first seeking to understand her brother's mental illness, trying to get an accurate diagnosis, and grappling with the possibility that she may be responsible for her brother's care. She said, "I went by myself in the public library and sat with a stack of books to read everything that I could about schizophrenia. . . . I spent a lot of time wondering about how or whether or not to tell other people. I learned at the time that the average onset for men is between the ages of eighteen and twenty-two, and for women, it is twenty-four to twenty-nine. I was twenty-four years old at the time I was reading about all of this." She talked about her experience of dating people and wondering, "At what moment do I trust this person to say that if you see me start to go crazy, you may have to tell me and help me recognize this. Can I trust this person enough? When you date people, do you ask or say, 'You may not want to have kids with me because of my family history'?"

Siblings also identified how their childhood relationships and later caregiving responsibilities shaped their own sense of mutuality, agency, self-esteem, health, and well-being. They related how much they supported each other, especially during important life transitions. Additionally, they talked about how, as difficult as the context can often make it to be a caregiver, being responsible for a sibling with serious mental illness makes them a better person and enriches their own understanding of self-giving love and God's care.

"I Could Not . . . Officiate at a Table Where My Baptized Sister Was Not Welcome."

A conversation I had with Deborah was particularly memorable because she reflected the many ways that she and her sister, Ann, care for each other. Ann was born with physical disabilities and developmental delays. These sisters have always had a good relationship and supported one another through important life transitions. As adults, Deborah became a legal guardian for Ann after both of their parents died in order to ensure that her sister had adequate support. Deborah also reflected on a time when her church made it more difficult to show her love for her sister by including her in a special service of worship.

Deborah is a Presbyterian pastor who was ordained in the 1970s in the Presbyterian Church USA and planned to serve communion during her ordination service. What is distinct about this story is that at that time, only those who had been baptized and confirmed were permitted to receive communion. Ann cannot read or write, tell time, and so on, so she was not allowed to participate in the confirmation process. It wasn't until the 1990s that mainstreaming in education and the church became more common. However, Ann, like the rest of the family, had been in church virtually every Sunday of her life.

Celebrating communion is not unusual at ordinations, and oftentimes, the newly ordained pastor presides over the table for the first time. Families and special friends or mentors are frequently included in the service. Deborah wanted to invite Ann to play a leadership role in the service. She remembered, "I was to celebrate the sacrament at my ordination but could not in good conscience officiate at a table where my baptized sister was not welcome." She asked her pastors "if there was anything [they] could do about the situation."

There was some provision for an exception if a minister and ruling elder "examined" the candidate and then recommended her to the session. In other words, Ann had to pass a test in order to be able to take communion with the rest of her family and the congregation. A conversation with the minister and an elder was arranged. Deborah sat in on the conversation in order to make her sister more comfortable and to help "translate" if Ann's speech was difficult to understand.

The minister asked, "Do you know who God is?"

Ann responded, "Yes, God made everything. But He didn't let the animals talk because it would be too noisy!"

The elder asked her, "Do you know who Jesus Christ is?"

"Yes," she said. "He is God's boy. They were very mean to him and hurt him. But it is OK now. God fixed it."

She was then asked if she knew who the Holy Spirit was. After a moment's reflection, Ann truthfully responded, "Not really; I never did quite get that part."

At the time, Deborah thought, "Pneumatology is pretty unclear to me too, and I have a PhD in theology!" In any event, Ann was permitted to receive communion. But that is not to suggest that receiving communion meant that all aspects of community life immediately opened up to her.

Deborah and Ann's story reminds us of the way Christian theology has been used to discriminate against people with intellectual disabilities and divide families. Historically, Christian theologians and religious leaders have connected the concept of human dignity to our creation in the image of God. Taking into account neurodiversity, theological language needs to name, and Christian rituals should affirm, a much richer and more textured understanding of human beings and how our creation reflects many images of God—*imagines Dei*.

"My Brother Crept in on My Individualism."

Dorothy admitted she struggles with Christian concepts of self-sacrifice when thinking about her life with Peter and her role as caregiver for him:

"There was a moment in my life that it felt deeply sacrificial to me, but when I think about certain instances in my life with my brother, [I see that caregiving] has also enhanced my sense of God's providence. If you sat me down when I was twenty [and said] that 'this is something you are going to do,' I wouldn't have believed it. But God has given me what I have needed at every stage."

Dorothy has learned to balance the concept of self-sacrificial love with the common good: "I come back again and again to the common good. To me, my shorthand definition of the common good is 'the good of all and the good of each.' I think it might be possible that we can say something about sacrifice and at the same time balance it with an understanding of the common good, which also requires determining or rightly ordering all of the goods. I know I wouldn't be the person I am today without my brother."

As an example, she pointed to how her brother helps her extend the boundaries of her own world: "It is very common for us to go shopping together, and my brother often stands outside the store smoking and talks with other people on the street. He always invites me to share with others. . . . What a gift that my brother crept in on my individualism and interrupted the way our jobs and economy demand efficiency." Dorothy's brother has lived with her for nearly twenty years. After all that time, she said, "I realize that I can't really be flourishing unless I am helping Peter to be his best."

Another sibling named Grace shared similar reflections about life with her brother Will. Grace is now fifty years old and lived away from her family for many years as she was building her own career. She returned to help her parents when Will experienced a psychotic episode and was hospitalized in acute care. Through the struggle that followed, Grace said she realized that her "story will never be inseparable from [her] brother or from God." She continued, "None of us are truly inseparable from each other and God—we belong to each other as one body."

———

The stories told by these individuals and families raise many questions about the origins of the stigma and shame associated with serious mental illness and what has shaped social attitudes and biases in the United States. Siblings whom I interviewed confirmed just how common it is for families who struggle with serious mental illness to conceal the problems they are facing out of fear of how others might perceive them. I also resonate with reflections made by many siblings about how the chaos and strangeness of their households took them by surprise. Remember Adair's observation that she didn't recognize how different her family life was from her peers' until she was about twelve years old and then had to seek the language that would help her name and describe her own experiences.

At some point in the lives of most siblings of people with serious mental illness, the silence and stigma becomes too great a burden to bear. Keeping all of the stories told in the last two chapters in mind, I will now provide a brief overview of the history of the treatment of people with mental illness in the United States and discuss why so many parents and siblings fear that their family member who struggles with mental illness may be forced into poverty. This history and description of the current situation will make clear that transforming these circumstances in which these families care for each other will require more than programmatic development. Disrupting the binary that divides able-bodied people from those with disabilities requires deepening our understanding of how the concept of disability is used to justify discrimination as well as learning more about varieties of human behavior. My aim in the next two chapters is to focus on pivotal moments in the history of madness in the United States and to provide enough detail to help us consider together new ways of claiming our humanity and speaking about God and dutiful love that are empowering for individuals, families, and other caregivers. I will also point out places where the social fabric of care is worn out, threadbare, or simply nonexistent so that we can work together to advocate for life-provisioning change for all those affected by serious mental illness.

PART II

History and Current Circumstances

A Brief Overview of the Treatment of People with Serious Mental Illness in the US Context

But truth is the highest consideration. *I tell what I have seen*—painful and as shocking as the details often are—that from them you may feel more deeply the imperative obligation which lies upon you to prevent the possibility of a repetition or continuance of such outrages upon humanity. If I inflict pain upon you, and move you to horror, it is to acquaint you with suffering which you have the power to alleviate, and make you hasten to the relief of the victims of legalized barbarity.

—Dorothea Dix, *Testimony before the Legislature of Massachusetts*

The treatment of mental illness from the very beginning of the North American experiment reflected Western European attitudes and approaches. This chapter considers the concept of disability brought to North America by European colonizers and how that frames early approaches to treatment for people with serious mental illnesses. John Winthrop preached his well-known sermon, "A Model of Christian Charity," in 1630 to other settlers of the Massachusetts Bay colony. The colonist's main mission was to restore the church by building a new society. Winthrop affirmed the variety and difference of all of God's "creatures, and the glory of His power in ordering all these differences."[1] In the seventeenth century, theology, philosophy, and what we now recognize as rudimentary medical science had a more porous relationship than they do today. Clergy served as spiritual leaders and also provided medical advice in the colonies. Mental and physical health could be seen as signs of God's blessing. It was also not uncommon to connect madness and melancholia to spiritual distress. As the colonies grew, advances in science and medicine offered new explanations for the causes of mental illness. Medical science emerged as a somewhat distinct field of inquiry by the end of the eighteenth century. Religious leaders, laypersons, and theologians gradually accepted medical theories and treatment of mental illness and began to strip away the theological terminology once used to explain its causes.

From the 1600s through the push toward deinstitutionalization in the 1950s, people with mental illness were, for the most part, associated with moral corruption and viewed as abnormalities, as weak, and as less than human. Healing, as opposed to empowerment, was understood as the restoration to an ideal state of mind, and social isolation was thought to create the best conditions for treatment. Within this context, Christian duty was primarily defined in terms of compassion, mercy, and providing treatment for charity cases. Jay Timothy Dolmage, a scholar in disability studies and activist, observes that "the body of history has been shaped to look like an idealized human body: proportional, inviolable, autonomous, upright, forward facing (white and masculine). But if you find the *rhetorical* body, you find tension, trial, and trouble."[2] My overview will primarily tell the story of how those considered healthy and normal shaped the lives and treatment of people with psychiatric disability. I will also be looking for noteworthy challenges to the stigmatization of people with mental illness made by family members, people of faith, and survivors of asylums or psychiatric hospitals.

This brief overview of history that leads into the twentieth century will be important for siblings and other family members to explain the marginalization of people with serious mental illness and the scarcity of resources available to families. Several of the siblings whom I interviewed grew up between the 1950s and 1970s, just after the APA published the first edition of the *Diagnostic and Statistical Manual of Mental Disorders* (DSM) and as the movement for deinstitutionalization gained force.

Their lives were directly affected by the shift from state-supported facilities to community-based mechanisms for care. Deinstitutionalization was intended to be empowering. Despite good intentions, however, it left many individuals and families to navigate a complex mental health system and without enough support to plan for lifelong care.

The Emergence of Reason's Other

Understanding the treatment of people with serious mental illness in the US context requires reviewing an earlier era and the formation of Western European attitudes toward disability—and more specifically, mental impairment—that would be brought to North America through the process of colonization. Historically, the first time we see realistic representations of disability in Western art and literature is in the late fifteenth century as the individual and reason become central to social and political thought in Europe. Tim Stainton, a historian and professor of social work, writes, "As the individual and his reason re-emerge as the central focus of social and political discourse, so too does the disabled subject, reason's other. . . . More importantly, we see the specific disabled subject as the metaphorical site of folly and the imaginary."[3]

A ship was a common metaphor for madmen and fools used in literature and art and related to the practice of communities entrusting some people with mental illness to sailors. They were literally set adrift on "the Ship of Fools, a strange 'drunken boat' that glides along the calm rivers of the Rhineland and the Flemish canals."[4] French philosopher Michel Foucault believed that journey was highly symbolic. Hieronymus Bosch's painting *The Ship of Fools* (1500) illustrates Foucault's claims. It is one of the most well-known depictions of a fool wearing a cap with bells. Foucault suggests that in these images, madness ceases to be at the limits of the world and becomes "an eschatological figure. . . . Oblivion falls upon the world navigated by the free slaves of the Ship of Fools."[5]

Policies to Protect the Body Politic
and the Body of Christ

Significant changes were enacted in official state policy by the late fifteenth century in Western Europe that were intended to protect the boundaries of both the church and nation-states. Medieval Christians, both Catholics and Protestants, thought of the church and society as bodies—the body of Christ and the body politic. By this time, Europeans had a great deal of experience with infectious diseases, most notably leprosy and the bubonic plague. The metaphors of the body politic and the body of Christ thus took on special meaning for people living with a recent memory of epidemic diseases.

Historian Nicholas Terpstra identifies the body as a metaphor in medieval thought with "different linked dimensions: the social Body of Christians (*Corpus Christianum*) drew ultimately on the spiritual Body of Christ (*Corpus Christi*)."[6] The main objective of the leaders of church and state became keeping the body of Christ and the body politic whole and well. They drew on medical language to sharpen their ideas and policies. Threats to the body were perceived as part of a cosmic struggle between good and evil, which fit within a particular reading of the biblical narrative. These shifts in thought and perception are evident in language and art.

Sickness and disease took on a moralistic meaning.[7] For example, the earliest usage of the term *pestilent* recorded in the *Oxford English Dictionary* was in 1398 and referred to plague or an epidemic of infectious disease. By 1425, the word was associated specifically with people or things that were "harmful or dangerous to religious, moral or social order."[8]

In connection, the metaphor of the body and the concept of the monster that was deeply rooted in ancient mythology began to figure prominently in art. Monsters represented otherness—the unknowable and mysterious—as both sacred and profane. Art historians Sherry Lindquist and Asa Simon Mittman emphasize that monsters in the Middle Ages depict bodies that "defy European notions of normality, bodily integrity, and the perceived limits of human nature."[9] Medieval artists drew on ancient writings about monsters to illustrate the demarcation between social and regional boundaries and to symbolically promote particular forms of interaction. The monstrous imagery associated with members of socially disadvantaged groups suggested their "subhuman" or threatening status.[10] Historians argue that "the monstrous is constitutive of both bodies that matter (humans, Christians, saints, historical figures, gendered subjects, and Christ) and, ostensibly, bodies that do not (animals, non-Christians, demons, fantastical creatures, and portentous freaks)."[11] Whole groups of outsiders were demonized, such as people with mental and physical impairments, Jews, Muslims, witches, and people from regions that Western Europeans associated with "lesser peoples."

Members of these groups were seen as pollutants and sources of contagion that could bring God's wrath upon the Christian community in the form of plagues and natural disasters. If infection threatened the body, then it had to be treated, contained, or completely removed. In terms of state policies, enclosure, containment, and exile were embraced as the means to keep the body healthy and well. Different types of enclosures were used in the Middle Ages to protect and purify the body politic and the body of Christ by keeping diverse groups of people "behind secure walls."[12] Containment held spiritual ramifications and preserved the wealth of particular Christians. These shifts in thought, perception, and policy lead Terpstra to suggest that the beginning of the era of Reformation should be marked with the expulsion of Jews from Spain in 1492 rather than the tacking of the *Ninety-Five Theses* by Martin Luther on a door of a church in Wittenberg.

Confinement as the Primary Means to Contain and Control

By the sixteenth century, political and religious forces coalesced to prompt a population shift toward urban centers, creating a rift in the feudal system. In the Catholic city of Paris, historians report that more than 30 percent of its population of about one hundred thousand citizens were beggars. Leprosariums were converted into institutions for the indigent, some of whom were also mentally ill. Foucault observed that thousands of

France's undesirables—petty criminals, prostitutes, homeless, and the insane—were institutionalized in an attempt to make society more rational and efficient. Confinement houses and asylums became widely accepted in the West as the solution to madness and melancholia when families did not have the means or ability to care for their kin.

Colonial Calvinists Connect Mental Illness with Spiritual Distress

These ideas about ensuring the health and wellness of the body politic and body of Christ traveled with the colonists to North America. Early on, colonists generally tolerated those considered insane as long as they were not seen as threatening the order within the community.[13] Throughout the colonies, people with mental illness who could not be cared for by their families were boarded with others.

Colonists who identified themselves as Calvinists understood all of creation to be subject to God's sovereignty—including rainbows, storms, earthquakes, deadly fires, and physical abnormalities. Their clergy rarely separated sickness and theology. Some directly linked physical and mental illness to sin, and health and prosperity could be seen as signs of God's favor. Sometimes sickness was understood as a trial to endure. Thus mental illness was connected with spiritual distress, and recommendations for cures incorporated natural and faith-based remedies.

Additionally, colonists brought with them from Europe the tradition of witch hunting. Those possessed by demons were culpable for their madness because they were believed to have sold their souls to the devil for their own gain. This view also lends itself to emphasizing human agency and responsibility to overcome madness without incorporating the reality of the lived experience of such ailments. At that time, it was considered appropriate to shackle or beat people who were believed to be possessed by demons. Nonnormative behaviors also sometimes brought expulsion or execution by drowning, burning, or hanging. The Salem witch trials, between 1691 and 1692, are the best-known example. Nineteen people were executed, two more died in jail, and one died from torture. The history here is more complex than often remembered. The trials could be seen as a possible consequence of the melding of medical and spiritual explanations for behavioral differences. New England Puritan minister Cotton Mather played a central role in the Salem witch trials even though he was not directly involved in the proceedings and later repented of his role in publicizing them. Mather was a pastor, theologian, and lay medical student. His writings show the mindset of colonists toward madness and also the way in which they blended theological and medical approaches to the treatment of disease.

Like other colonial Calvinists, Mather believed that illness could fulfill a spiritual role and serve as an aspect of both personal and social conversion to a more divinely ordered reality. Mather was a prolific author and published several works that addressed demon possession, madness, and melancholia. *The Angel of Bethesda* (1724), a book written for physicians and clergy, included chapters on "Madness" and "Melancholy." Mather wrote, "You may often see Cause to Suspect, that the *Spiritual Troubles of* your *Melancholicks* are not of such an *Original* [sin] as is pretended for. If you trace them, you may perhaps find out, that some very intolerable *Vexation*, or some *Temporal Troubles*, begun their Uneasiness, and first raised that *Ulcer* in their Minds."[14]

As the populations of colonial communities grew and became more organized, the presence of mental illness was more visible, and leaders looked to Western Europe for approaches to treatment. Communities opened hospitals, asylums, and workhouses for dependent citizens, institutions that set the stage for care within the US context for around two hundred years. Pennsylvania Hospital was the first to be established in 1751 in Philadelphia, the fastest-growing city in the colonies. The hospital maintained special provisions for "lunatics." Other states followed suit, and specialized hospitals were created in Connecticut, Massachusetts, New York, Virginia, and South Carolina. Most of the beds in the Pennsylvania facility were designated for lunatics thought to be dangerous and disruptive. Hospital personnel at that time also thought it was rational to treat people with mental illness harshly. Cells for lunatics were not usually heated because of the prevalent belief that mentally ill people could not feel temperature differences. Other treatments included hot and cold showers (alternately), the shaving and blistering of scalps, bleeding and purging, and chaining by the ankle or waist to the wall of a cell.

New Scientific Theories and a Shift toward Humane Treatment

Several factors stimulated a shift toward the more humane treatment of people with mental illness in the late eighteenth and early nineteenth centuries. New scientific theories emerged from the work of European physicians and scholars trying to rescue the scientific study of mental disorders from traditions of witch hunting. In addition, physicians such as Philippe Pinel of France, Vincenzo Chiarugi of Italy, and Benjamin Rush of North America advanced the call for humane treatment within institutions, then called asylums. Philanthropists such as William Tuke in England provided support for building retreats to serve as alternatives to the old model asylums.

Benjamin Rush and the Turn toward Natural Causes of Mental Illness

Benjamin Rush was both a physician and a lay theologian. He was also one of the first US doctors to challenge the theological connection made between human sinfulness and mental illness. He entered into a broader debate among medical doctors, clergy, and laypersons, and from these conversations, many competing theories of the interrelation between the mind and human behavior developed. Historian Heather Vacek says that Rush's work represents a transitional moment in the field of psychiatry. Rush relied on scientific knowledge in an era when most physicians looked to both "medicine and morality to explain mental maladies."[15]

Rush paid particular attention to people whose madness led them to attempt or commit suicide and based his claims on observations he made of patients with mental disease at Pennsylvania Hospital. Rush "believed in 'faculty psychology,'" the prevailing idea that humans were born with faculties of the mind that subserved the emotions, thought, and behavior.[16] He argued against earlier medical theories that rooted the source of disease in the balance of the body's fluids or in passions, yet he held on to treatments such as bloodletting. In 1812, Rush published *Medical Inquiries and Observations upon the Diseases of the Mind*, the first US textbook in psychiatry, in which he attributed the causes of insanity to abnormal blood flow. After the publication of this work, many clergy turned toward medicine for insights into mental illness. In addition, tension grew between clinicians, who derived knowledge through observation of the sick, and anatomists, who looked for physical sources of mental illness. It was not until the twentieth century that medical explanations for mental illness fully usurped theological and moral ones. But Rush's work helped stimulate a move toward institutionalized care within asylums that would incorporate moral treatment.

The Perception That Insanity Is on the Rise

Another reason for the shift toward institutionalized care had to do with the perception that insanity was growing. Insanity captured the public's attention and became an ever-present theme in popular literature of the time as people sought to understand the causes. Some argued that rapid industrialization and urbanization caused stress, saying city life itself contributed to the increasing numbers of those considered insane. Others blamed immigrants, particularly Irish Catholics, as "a major cause of increasing insanity."[17] Some suggested insanity was "part and parcel of poverty."[18] Before the Civil War, slaveholders defended slavery as a legitimate and compassionate institution because the conditions of freedom would drive slaves insane. For example, John C. Calhoun, a former vice president and US Senator, said, "The African is incapable of self-care and sinks into lunacy under the burden of freedom. It is mercy to give him the guardianship and protection from mental death."[19] These ideas reflected a prominent belief from the Victorian era—namely, that bodies mark the boundary between chaos and meaningless and order and holiness. Thus Victorian notions of industriousness and white upper- and middle-class norms were standardized and marketed as the most ideal and efficient for Western societies in the midst of modernization.[20]

Pseudoscience and Freak Shows Reinforce Stigma

Alongside the advances in medical knowledge, the development of humane treatment, and fears that insanity was on the rise, pseudosciences such as phrenology and the creation and success of a new form of entertainment known as the freak show gained popularity. "Extraordinary" bodies—those considered abnormal, different, deformed, and disabled—were presented as visible contrasts to Victorian notions of industriousness and white middle-class norms.

Phrenology

Phrenology was grounded in the theories of Franz Gall and brought to the United States by Johann Spurzheim. The intention of this pseudoscience was to liberate concepts of the mind from faith-oriented ideas and focus on scientific explanations of mental capacities and ailments. Phrenologists believed they could locate the origins of difference, disease, and deformity by studying the contours of the human cranium and other physical features. Some of Gall's earliest studies were of inmates in jails and lunatic asylums. Church authorities in his home country of Austria resisted Gall's theories, but their disapproval only increased public interest and prompted him to leave Europe to lecture in the United States.

As ridiculous and dangerous as phrenology sounds in the twenty-first century, it gained a tremendous following. Several books and almanacs written by phrenologists became international best sellers. At the height of phrenology's popularity in the United States, employers asked for character references from phrenologists. Some superintendents of mental hospitals incorporated phrenology into their care for patients. For example, Amariah Brigham, one of the founding members of the Association of Medical Superintendents of American Institutions for the Insane, which eventually became the APA, incorporated phrenology into his work. The popular tide turned against phrenology by 1860, and the pseudoscience was discredited for being used to support slavery and notions of a superior race.

Freak Shows

Freak shows increased in popularity in the 1840s and remained an entertainment attraction until about 1940. Some historians argue that the concept of the "freak" was created and marketed to make visible the contrast between people who fit the culturally acceptable able-bodied and white middle-class norms and those with bodies and minds that couldn't fit into these molds. Historian Rosemarie Garland Thomson contends, "Mechanized practices such as standardization, mass production, and interchangeable parts promoted sameness of form as a cultural value and made singularity in both products and bodies seem deviant."[21] It became socially acceptable to attend the "formally organized exhibition of people with alleged physical, mental, or behavioral difference at circuses, fairs, carnivals, and other amusement venues."[22] Those put on display were marked on billboards and flyers as "human oddities," "cultural exotics," "armless and legless wonders," "fat people," "giants," and so on. Parallels can be drawn between the "enfreakment" of people with mental and physical impairments and Africans, immigrants, and people living in poverty. All those marketed as "human oddities" were seen as socially disruptive, needing to be controlled and contained, and associated with incivility and the total lack of reason.

Even as these cultural dynamics continued to shape social attitudes toward people with mental and physical differences, medical professionals increasingly focused on treating mental illness as primarily a medical concern rather than a social problem. During this same period, we see little evidence of churches acting to empower people with mental illness or so-called disabling conditions to speak out for themselves. Some churches did advocate for state-supported asylums. But they adopted primarily a charitable approach to this advocacy in an effort to improve the conditions of people they considered spiritually impoverished.

Pioneering a More Humane and Moral Treatment

Throughout the nineteenth century, there were many who believed that people with mental illness deserved to be treated harshly, but some drew on advances in psychology and psychiatry as well as moral arguments to advocate for a more humane approach to treatment and care. French physician Pinel pioneered an approach to care for people with mental illness known as *traitment moral* (moral treatment). Moral treatment named a new disposition of care as well as a set of techniques. Two basic principles informed Pinel's concept: First, mental disorders affected an individual's moral faculties without completely overwhelming their sense of reason. Second, intervention and treatment should uphold the sense of dignity of the individual and be based on the promotion of hope and kindness. Some scholars argue that peer support practices can be traced back to Pinel's approach and the partnership he developed with Jean-Baptiste Pussin, the governor of Bicêtre Hospital in France. One of their first actions was to free inmates from their chains and then hire convalescing patients to help treat their peers.[23]

Tuke was a Quaker leader who founded the York Retreat in England to counter the harshness of some other asylums and practices of confinement. He took a more educational and disciplinary approach.[24] The staff at York Retreat assumed that the inner light or "divine spark" within each resident was never fully distinguished. Faith and spirituality were believed to be positive and civilizing influences within his approach to humane treatment. In the early 1800s, a series of hospitals based on the York Retreat example opened in the United States.

Another important reformer is Dorothea Dix. Dix earned a reputation as a reformer and advocate when she began traveling in 1836, and throughout the rest of her life, she covered thousands of miles as she visited county jails, state prisons, poorhouses, and other institutions in the United States and Europe. During her visits, she chronicled the treatment of the insane and reported to state and federal legislatures the horrific, unsanitary conditions in which they were forced to live. Prisons were largely unregulated and lacked proper sanitation. Dix documented accounts of prisoners being flogged, starved, chained, physically and sexually abused, and left naked without heat or sanitation.

Advocacy, for Dix, became a sacred cause. Growing up in a family affected by mental illness fueled her passion to work for change. Ultimately, she galvanized a movement as she testified before state legislatures and in Washington, DC. She advocated for state-supported asylums that would offer an institutionalized model of care where people with mental illness would be treated by a professional and trained staff. Asylums would offer three to four months of "moral therapy" that Dix and others at the time believed could restore patients to an ideal state of mind. The key to recovery in this approach rested in the removal of mentally imbalanced people from the stress of big-city life. Inmates were required to live according to routines established by the superintendent, which incorporated religious exercises, games, and rest.

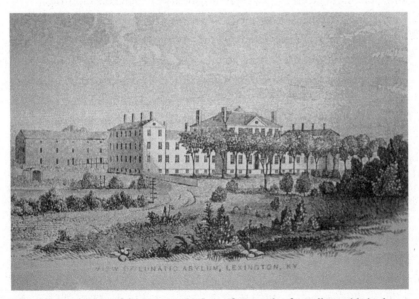

Figure 3.1 Drawing of the Lunatic Asylum of Kentucky, formally established in 1821 and opened in 1824. Similar asylums were built all across the nation. Image created by Clay Lancaster. Clay Lancaster Slide Collection. University of Kentucky Special Collections.

Dix played a decisive role in founding or expanding more than thirty asylums. Like many other advocates in her day, she voiced concerns on behalf of people with mental illness and urged compassion and charity for their cause but fell short of creating spaces that would empower them to give voice to their own concerns and experiences.

Over time, asylums earned a reputation for mistreating patients and repeated many of the same mistakes made in previous eras due to several factors. Asylums were built in rural areas to create a restful environment, but that isolation left some residents without family support. Moral treatment required extensive and costly training, and many state legislatures were reluctant to invest large sums of money in people with mental illness. After the Civil War, asylum populations grew, incorporating many freed slaves, veterans suffering "soldier's heart," and immigrants. Some asylums became like minicities, including factories or other forms of labor in order for residents to have work. In some cases, this re-created the stratification and challenges faced by people living in large urban communities.

Other theories and treatments were vying for respectability in the last quarter of the nineteenth century, including some that moved outside institutional settings. Sigmund Freud theorized that early childhood experiences shaped the self and personality. His theories gained prominence and turned doctors' attention to the unconscious mind. Freud began to associate religion with hysteria and neurosis rather than emphasizing its positive influences. Growth in the fields of psychology and psychiatry was strong, incorporating significant work done by neurologist and psychiatrist Wilhelm Griesinger, who postulated that mental illness was a disease of the brain; psychiatrist Wilhelm Wundt, who began to separate psychology from philosophy; and anthropologist Francis Galton, who conducted studies in human behavior and genetics. Alongside the expansion in these fields, the number of state facilities for people with mental illness increased through the middle of the twentieth century; more than half a million people resided in such institutions in the United States by the mid-1950s.

Eugenics Cast in Its Time as a Movement for the "Betterment of the Human Race"

Psychological causes and medical cures usurped supernatural and religious ones within the first third of the twentieth century. Liberal clergy influenced by higher criticism of the Bible yielded authority regarding mental health issues, handed things over to medical professionals, and in many ways ignored the subject of insanity. By the mid-1920s, the medical community reached some consensus that mental illness was organic and that religious leaders, pastors, and students of theology would waste their time by trying to discern religious or theological meaning from the experience. Psychiatrists in Europe and the United States began to adopt new perspectives about the genetic causes of mental illness that were influenced by social Darwinism and genetic determinism.

Social Darwinism gained popularity between the 1880s and the 1930s. This theory applied the idea of survival of the fittest to the social order. Eugenics was able to gain significant influence, as it partnered well with social Darwinist theory. The term *eugenics* was first coined in the late 1800s by Francis Galton, half-cousin to Charles Darwin, and literally means "to be born well." Galton analyzed the characteristics of the British upper class and associated superior intellect with social elites. He concluded that this trait was hereditary.

In the United States, the eugenics movement took root in the early 1900s. It was first advanced by biologist Charles Davenport and an educator named Harry Laughlin. Oil tycoon and philanthropist John D. Rockefeller was among other prominent funders of eugenics research.

Eugenicists favored immigration laws excluding Asians, nonwhites, and Jews and limited quotas set for eastern and southern European immigrants. Jay Dolmage links the rhetoric surrounding immigration to eugenics in his book *Disabled upon Arrival: Eugenics, Immigration, and the Construction of Race and Disability*. He argues that restrictive immigration policies in the United States have never really been "fully about immigration. Simply: immigration has been about creating a dominant normative identity; it has been about translating written and spoken and visual arguments about the value of bodies into action, mapping them onto other, bigger ideas like continents."[25] Ellis Island, a major port of entry into the United States from 1890 to 1925, "became a key laboratory and operating theater for American eugenics."[26] Racist and ableist ideologies were employed to identify and stigmatize "undesirable" people with abnormality, illness, physical disability, insanity, and criminality.

Eugenicists also advocated for laws to prevent people with mental illness and learning disabilities from marrying. Indiana, Laughlin's home state, passed the first compulsory sterilization laws in 1907 and was considered to be on the cutting edge of Progressive reforms. Eugenicists argued for sterilization on the basis that "the mentally deficient" were "a serious menace to all civilization," and "morons were reproducing more rapidly than persons of sound intelligence."[27] Regulating fertility would strengthen families and the nation, and the most compassionate response was to stop "feeble-minded persons" from reproducing for the sake of the betterment of society.

Eugenics struck a chord with many mainline Protestants, especially its emphasis on "chosenness," which echoed in Calvinist theology. A strong belief pervading mainline denominations was that Anglo-Saxon Protestants were the standard-bearers of Christianity and civilization in the United States. Social Gospelers—including Washington Gladden, Harry Emerson Fosdick, Shailer Mathews, and Walter Rauschenbusch—attempted to reconcile Christianity with contemporary reform movements, science among them. Many social gospelers promoted eugenics. Historian Christine Rosen observes, "It is easy to see why ministers of the Social Gospel would find eugenics appealing. The two movements shared certain assumptions. Salvation for Social Gospelers was a social matter; social redemption was as much a part of salvation as one's own personal redemption. In a similar vein, eugenicists argued that heredity should be a social matter, and they too supported intervention and reform to guarantee the preservation of the race. Both groups appealed to society's social conscience in the interest of reform."[28] Some congregations created lending libraries to promote eugenics literature. Other organizations, such as the American Eugenics Society, sponsored sermon contests to promote the biblical foundation for eugenics and published "A Eugenics Catechism." Vacek writes, "In the hands of some,

Jesus' parables regarding the kingdom of God swiftly became parables for the eugenic separation of human wheat from human chaff."[29] Some eugenicists thought of eugenics as a religion with guarding the "germ plasm" as a form of stewardship.

A few movements opposed eugenics, including grassroots Catholic and conservative Christian ones. The Vatican, however, did not weigh in on eugenics until 1930 in Pope Pius IX's encyclical on Christian marriage, *Casti Connubii*, which focused on birth control but also renounced eugenics. Regrettably, most mainline denominations have still not apologized for their support of eugenics and involuntary sterilization policies related to this pseudoscience. I am aware of only one mainline denomination, the United Methodist Church, that officially apologized for supporting eugenics in a statement calling for "An Apology for Support of Eugenics," which was passed by their general conference in 2008.

By 1933, forty-eight US states had sterilization laws preventing certain individuals from "breeding." From 1907 to the mid-1950s, 65,000 people were involuntarily sterilized in the United States; more than a third of them resided in mental hospitals. US sterilization laws were widely copied in Europe. In 1933, when Hitler was promoted into a position of power, Germany passed a comprehensive sterilization policy. Between 1933 and 1939, 375,000 Germans were involuntarily sterilized. World War II was a kind of reckoning for the US eugenics movements, but twenty-seven US states kept sterilization laws on the books until 1956. The last mandatory sterilization in the United States was in 1981 in the state of Oregon.

After World War I, a variety of other medical treatments that were considered "advances" were used in asylums. Physicians put patients into a low blood sugar coma during insulin coma therapy because they believed large fluctuations in insulin levels could alter the function of the brain. Other treatments included malaria fever therapy, metrazol shock, electroconvulsive shock therapy, the lobotomy procedure, sterilization, and clitoridectomy.

Due to overcrowding in mental institutions, the frontal lobotomy was introduced in 1935. This surgery gained popularity in the United States, especially when Walter Jackson Freeman II simplified the procedure.[30] It was seen as a treatment that made patients easier to handle. In addition to the use of the lobotomy procedure, federal funding–sponsored programs in hospitals and clinics used involuntary sterilization to limit the growth of "undesirable" populations, including immigrants, people of color, people in poverty, single mothers, and people with mental and physical impairments. Doctors also subjected patients to other unnecessary procedures in addition to the lobotomy. At Stockton State Hospital in California, five women ranging in ages from twenty-nine to forty-nine underwent both lobotomy and clitoridectomy between 1947 and 1950.[31]

An Alternative Approach to Caregiving: "Living Human Documents"

In hindsight, it is difficult to understand how such theories and treatments could be promoted for the "betterment of the human race" when they denied the humanity and agency of people with mental impairments and illnesses. An alternative approach at the time was created as a result of the firsthand experiences of such treatments. In 1920, Anton Boisen's family committed him to Boston Psychopathic Hospital due to the psychotic episodes he was experiencing. Boisen was also a congregational minister. While at the hospital, he developed the hypothesis that mental illness was caused by something that upset the foundation on which the patient's reasoning was based. He concluded after his release that he wanted to provide much-needed pastoral care to people with mental illness.

Boisen identified as problematic many approaches to mental illness and mental health in the early twentieth century. Pastors and priests ceded their religious authority and much of the influence of faith communities to medical professionals. Religious leaders were too distracted by the fundamentalist-modernist controversy to address the desperate need for care for people with mental illness. He raked both fundamentalists and liberals over the coals for different reasons: Fundamentalists had "no clear idea of what salvation means nor of what people need to be saved from."[32] Liberals supplied "neither treatment nor diagnosis."[33] Most of the medical community believed that mental illness was organic and that it would be a waste of time for theological students to try to discern religious or theological meaning in the treatment of patients. Academic theologians also largely ignored the importance of people as "living human documents" and the theologies that emerged from their experiences. Theological education largely focused on scholarly literature. Boisen wanted to turn the attention of pastors, priests, and theologians toward reading "human documents with the same reverence, respect, and depth with which one using modern hermeneutical method reads biblical texts."[34]

In his mind, the seminaries were largely responsible for ceding religious authority to medical professionals. Boisen did not think theology should just be an academic enterprise; it required encounters with other human beings in the spirit of what he called "cooperative" or "interdisciplinary" inquiry. He was particularly critical of theologians such as Reinhold Niebuhr. Niebuhr's "empirical studies of human nature are very limited," Boisen wrote. "His discussion of the problem of sin leaves one with the impression that his standpoint is not that of one who is trying sympathetically to understand the frailties and misbehavior of men, but rather than of one who looks upon them from the standpoint of the Almighty and finds in pride the greatest of all sins."[35] Boisen's own method incorporated case study analysis and theological reflection on lived human experience.

Dr. Richard Cabot, a medical physician and reformer during this era, developed a partnership with Boisen to found the first program in clinical pastoral education (CPE). Working together with other pastoral theologians, they identified a need for "'liaison officers' between medical workers in psychiatry, with their already advanced knowledge, and religious workers at large."[36] CPE introduced a collaborative approach between medical professionals and clergy and created a place for health and welfare institutions to play a formative role within theological education.

For a brief period after World War II, churches directed their attention toward mental health, and support for mental health initiatives grew. This surge of interest related to soldiers returning from war with what was called at that time combat stress reaction or "battle fatigue." This interest was driven in part by reports coming from conscientious objectors who were doing alternative service in mental hospitals. New efforts for collaboration between medical and religious professionals were accompanied by "new wartime insights about mental distress, the popularization of psychoanalytic theories, national legislation of mental health provision, massive mid-century deinstitutionalization of mental hospitals, and the development of grassroots advocacy groups in support of sufferers."[37] One of the most noted advocates in the medical field who took up Boisen's charge was Dr. Karl Menninger. Menninger viewed mental illness not as a perpetual state but rather as a way of behaving or functioning that affects all people at some point in their lives. His work helped reshape public perceptions, and he founded a private, innovative inpatient mental hospital from which he and other colleagues could launch training programs for mental health professionals.

Deinstitutionalization: Shifting the Burden of Care

By the mid-1940s, state institutions were publicly exposed for providing substandard care. Albert Q. Maisel published an article in *Life Magazine* entitled "Bedlam 1946" in which he compared state-sponsored asylums to concentration camps. Maisel reported on what he witnessed after visiting a number of state institutions and provided corroborating evidence from narratives written by about three thousand conscientious objectors or "conchies"—many Methodist, Quaker, Mennonite, and Brethren—who served state institutions in lieu of picking up arms. They gave testimony on behalf of hundreds of people being beaten and abused, thousands spending their days locked in "devices euphemistically called 'restraints,'" and hundreds confined to filthy isolation rooms without beds.[38] Moreover, Maisel found that asylums were overcrowded and underfunded, and residents were often being fed a starvation diet. His exposé, along with the testimony of many "conchies," stimulated reform.

The discovery of antipsychotic drugs in the 1950s strengthened the deinstitutionalization movement and dramatically changed the course of modern psychiatry. A serious push began within many countries, including the United States, to move away from institutionalized care for people with mental illness and toward community-based care and consumer empowerment. Additionally, in 1956, President Eisenhower signed into law an amendment to the Social Security Act to include state-funded social insurance benefits for people with disabilities.

These factors, along with the election of John F. Kennedy as president in 1960, spurred a new wave of change. One of JFK's eight siblings, Rosemary, had intellectual disabilities and then developed mental illness in her teen years. In 1941, doctors convinced her parents that a lobotomy could bring the promise of a cure. She was just twenty-three years old. The surgery dramatically altered the rest of her life, limiting her mobility, exacerbating her intellectual impairments, and leaving her without the ability to care for her own physical needs. The Kennedys were wealthy enough to pay for top-notch care for Rosemary in private hospitals and then later in a Catholic school for exceptional adults. However, their ability to support Rosemary in private facilities did not keep her completely out of the public eye. After John F. Kennedy won the presidential election, he and his sister Eunice did what many siblings would do: they made fixing the nation's broken mental health system central to their life's work.

In 1961, Kennedy convened two groups to address the problem and determine a solution: the President's Panel on Mental Retardation and the Interagency Committee on Mental Health. Eunice Kennedy Shriver became the lightning rod to address learning disabilities and differences. Shriver founded the Special Olympics in 1968. Some animosity existed between those who advocated for people with intellectual and developmental disabilities and those who advocated for individuals with serious mental illness. Proposals to create a better context to support people with intellectual disabilities and those with mental illness were made independent of each other and achieved varying levels of success.

Kennedy signed into law the Community Mental Health Centers (CMHC) Construction Act in 1963, shortly before he was assassinated. This act facilitated the closure of many state hospitals in the United States. Strict standards were passed regarding who could be committed to state hospitals. Only individuals who posed an imminent danger to themselves or others could be so committed. The first CMHC opened in 1966, but evidence suggests that patients were being released from state hospitals before the act was signed and while it was being debated. Many patients in state asylums who were thought to be stabilized by medications were released. Alarmingly, members of the committee who created the CMHC concept had ignored statistics that showed 75 percent of those housed in state hospitals had no families to which they could return or did not have families willing to accept them.

Federal funding was initially only secured for five years (later eight), and efforts on the federal level to create a new national mental health system bypassed leaders on the state and local levels, limiting collaboration, coordination, and communication. States also had differing levels of ability to pick up the funding of the CMHCs. When the CMHC Act was signed, the federal government intended to offer a declining level of support over a set period of time while states would increase their support of CMHCs. For example, the CMHCs were funded by the federal government 100 percent in the first year. In the second year, the act proposed that states take over 10 percent of the costs and increase the percentage of their support over the next few years. Unfortunately, poorer states could never adequately pick up their share of the funding.

In 1965, President Lyndon B. Johnson signed the Social Security Amendments Act, which created Medicare and Medicaid. Medicaid funded health care for low-income families and, in the case of mental health treatment, gave major impetus for the use of antipsychotic medications for the treatment of mental illness, but it did not pay for psychiatric hospitalization. As people were released from state-sponsored hospitals, beds designated for psychiatric care were eliminated, and many hospitals were closed. Thus when someone had a more severe episode of their mental illness, fewer options for care and for housing were available. States were forced to transfer many mental health patients into nursing homes. Since hospitalization for mental health issues was not always covered, some facilities recorded that patients were being treated for different conditions in order to access Medicare coverage. Several additional attempts were made by later presidential administrations to address gaps in insurance coverage for mental health care, to increase funding for Medicare and Medicaid coverage, and to address other problems created by deinstitutionalization, but the problem has never been fully resolved.[39]

To this day, serious mental illness is not treated the same as physical illness for a variety of reasons. The influence of the private insurance industry in the United States creates a distinctive context for mental and physical health care in comparison to other countries. State-funded social insurance programs for the purpose of assisting people with diagnosed disabilities have also always been debated. Questions are raised about the costs of funding the programs and about how to prove that a diagnosed disability prevents someone from working. As a result, modifications of state-funded programs are introduced. For example, Medicare and Medicaid were modified early on in 1972 by incorporating a provision related to health maintenance organizations (HMOs). This change reflects a larger public ideological battle regarding efficiencies created by private insurance, the role and responsibility of the state to provide social welfare and health care for all, and personal responsibility to control behaviors associated with mental illness.

Bringing the Point of This Chapter Home

Most importantly, for individuals and families, the shifts in attitudes and treatment and the movement toward deinstitutionalization in the United States directly impact their lives. Let me bring this chapter home by sharing the story of how these changes affected a family. Glenn, one of the siblings whom I interviewed, grew up in the late 1960s and early 1970s. He reflected on the complexity of planning for his brother's care. The nature of his brother's mental illness made it difficult even for their mother to understand. She was a nurse and had just enough medical knowledge to believe that she could help him recover. This belief was bolstered by her fundamentalist faith, which encouraged her to see everything as "black and white." I took that to mean that Glenn's brother was either restored to a state of mental health or sick. So times when he seemed better meant that they could return to some sense of a "normal" life. Glenn said,

> There hasn't been a good plan. It looks like he has the right doctors and the right community, but then something happens, and he doesn't

like it there and so he wants to leave. He has the freedom to leave, and he would just leave and take a taxi to my mom. He really hasn't had good care the whole time. He has been in some good places, but he has left those places. The process of dealing with a physical illness is a lot more clear cut than the process of dealing with a mental illness. With a physical illness, there is a clear-cut plan. Say you have a stroke; there is a plan in the hospital, and then you go and get physical therapy.

Glenn is well aware of the precarity of his brother's circumstances. But family relationships and his mother's emotions also often make navigating the mental health system even more challenging. One of the biggest fears Glenn and several other siblings expressed to me in our conversations is the difficulty of planning for lifelong care and the possibility that their brother or sister will end up living in extreme poverty or on the streets. The lack of social safety nets available makes these fears very realistic.

CHAPTER FOUR

Prescription for Poverty

At least jail is a free place to live.

—Neville

Almost anywhere you live in the world, unless you are born into an extremely wealthy family, a diagnosis of serious mental illness carries along with it a prescription for poverty and potential homelessness largely because of the stigma surrounding mental illness and the difficulty of accessing adequate mental health care. According to the World Health Organization (WHO), "An overwhelming majority of people with mental and psychosocial disabilities are living in poverty, poor physical health, and are subject to human rights violations."[1] Additionally, family caregivers, 60 percent of whom are women, remain largely unpaid, which impacts their own lives. One in four caregivers will face financial difficulties. Many work a second job, are forced to reduce their working hours, or must forgo income or benefits in order to keep up with their responsibilities.

Recent studies also suggest that the circumstances of living in poverty exacerbate mental illness.[2] Mental disorders such as depression are twice as frequent among people living in poverty because of hunger and poor nutrition, overcrowded housing, poor sanitation, lack of access to education, unemployment or underemployment, and worry about debt. People of the lowest socioeconomic status worldwide are eight times more likely to experience schizophrenia, a condition associated with high rates of unemployment, divorce, and potential homelessness. Impoverished people lack access to quality medical care, healthy foods that can contribute to emotional and physical well-being, educational opportunities for social advancement, and other costly support services. Wealth inequalities and the inability to meet one's own basic needs cultivate social anxiety.

In the United States, 29 percent of people with a diagnosed serious mental illness live in poverty, compared to 12 percent of people without a disability.[3] The US Department of Housing and Urban Development reported in 2015 that about one-third of all people who are homeless have an untreated mental illness. Today, county jails have become one of the nation's largest holding pens for people with serious mental illness, particularly those who cannot afford adequate health care coverage and often lack the extensive network of support required to navigate their circumstances. Despite this and other statistical evidence, it can be difficult for those who have not directly experienced the debilitating effects of serious mental illness and the brokenness of our mental health system to understand the causes of and correlation between poverty and mental illness.

Those causes are complex, and the issues are challenging to disentangle. This chapter explores a variety of factors that contribute to and cause poverty and the disproportionately high rates of unemployment, homelessness, and incarceration among people with serious mental illness. It also highlights the lack of support for families and caregivers. It is not possible here to discuss in full detail the complex public policy decisions in the United States that led to evaluating and providing significantly different levels of care for mental and physical health, so I have included a "Timeline of Significant Events Related to Policy Shifts, Treatment, and Attitudes toward Mental Illness from the Mid-twentieth Century to the Present" in the "Additional Resources" section at the end of this book. This reference shows key historical markers in the ever-declining cycle of care for people with psychiatric disability. However, my intention in this chapter is to help you and faith communities identify places where advocacy is needed and can make a difference for individuals and families affected by serious mental illness. I highlight three major systemic and structural causes of poverty among individuals with serious mental illness and their families: (1) health care policies intended to make mental health care more cost efficient, cost effective, and profitable; (2) limitations placed on disability benefits; and (3) disparities in the distribution of allocated resources for mental health care.

On a systemic and structural level, resources allocated for mental health care are far more limited than for physical health care even though treatment for a mental illness is incredibly costly. The well-intended but poorly planned deinstitutionalization movement in the United States that began in the 1950s damaged the fabric of care that existed on the state level and left individuals, families, and communities without the resources necessary to care for the most serious and chronic cases. The community mental health resources that were to be developed to support deinstitutionalized patients never materialized in any significant way. Assumptions about the legal competency of individuals with serious mental illness to determine their own fate reduced their access to the kind of supportive care, residences, and services that those with intellectual and developmental disabilities received. Moreover, social safety nets in the United States are far too small when considering the high cost of an individual's lifelong struggle with mental illness, unemployment, underemployment, and homelessness. Central to these systemic and structural issues is the inherent and embedded assumption that people with serious mental illness are somehow personally responsible for their health issues, can be cured if they want to badly enough, and have the potential to navigate the system and interact with others in their community the same way as their able-minded and able-bodied peers.

Policies Intended to Make Health Care More Efficient and Maximize Profits

For decades, US society has engaged in an invisible but tangible war over resources—financial, educational, and so on. Theologians, ethicists, philosophers, political scientists, economists, and journalists have paid a great deal of attention in recent years to the root causes of the increasing wealth divide in our nation and around the world. The root causes of poverty and the growing wealth divide parallel the increasing gap in access to mental health care. A political economic project known as neoliberalism began to gain traction in the United States in the 1970s. President Ronald Reagan and Prime Minister Margaret Thatcher are credited with leading the shift toward neoliberal economic policies in the 1980s, although economic historians cite the origins of this political economic project as early as 1947. For neoliberals, freedom and markets are synonymous. To paraphrase economist Philip Mirowski, when the market no longer gives you what you want, you have to capitulate to what the market wants. All areas of life improve when they become more market driven. In terms of physical and mental health care policy, this means that private insurers are seen as more efficient providers of care and more effective at controlling costs than a government plan.

US health care policies take a market-oriented approach that looks to increase cost-effectiveness, efficiency, and profitability to solve problems of access to and affordability of health care, including mental health care. The United States is "the only western industrialized nation that fails to provide universal coverage and the only nation where health care for the majority is financed by for-profit, minimally regulated health insurance companies."[4] When it comes to mental and physical impairments, the only way to make disabled minds and bodies profitable is by setting limits on care, shifting costs to government-funded agencies, and placing the burden on individuals and their families. Social and economic values embedded in health care rationing were brought into sharp relief during the COVID-19 pandemic as twenty-five states enacted policies that prioritized ventilators or other supports and pushed people with disabilities to the back of the line.[5] Those who are the least efficient and seen as unemployable, along with their families, live in the cross fire with few defenses. Frequently, they are submerged into poverty; forced into more efficient, institutionalized models of care; or provided with limited or no access to much-needed mental health care.

Experts on health care and economic policy argue that health care has always posed a bigger challenge than economic, transportation, or education policy for neoliberal theorists and politicians because of the failure of private markets to attend to health needs. The inability of laborers to care for themselves and their family members during bouts of illness and periods during which they were unable to work originally stimulated interest in sickness insurance and created programs like Medicare and Medicaid in the United States. Caring for sick bodies can be inefficient and is not always profitable, particularly when someone has a chronic illness. From 1972 until the passage of the Affordable Care Act (ACA) in 2010, social insurance provided by Medicare and Medicaid underwent a series of modifications that trended toward privatization. Medicare's framework was changed from a purely public insurance to a competitive market and placed a stronger emphasis on personal responsibility in order to increase cost-efficiency and preserve financial capital.

The privatization of health care became increasingly common under the Reagan administration, and due to changes in the way federal grants were offered for mental health care, state providers were forced to compete for funding with organizations providing for other public needs such as housing and food banks. State hospitals continued to eliminate beds or close, and nursing homes that could access Medicaid and Medicare funding increasingly became the dumping grounds for younger patients with chronic and severe mental illness.[6]

Several additional attempts have been made to improve the nation's mental health system, but many have been thwarted by private interests in health care and the insurance industry. Sheila Schuster, a licensed clinical psychologist and leading voice in advocacy regarding mental health policy, suggests that private insurance companies have always hidden behind the stigma associated with mental illness and used it to deny coverage and services. Insurance companies have argued that treatment for mental illness should be limited because of the difficulty in finding the right diagnosis and the challenge of measuring outcomes. They feared these were too easily open to abuse. Insurance companies have never offered the same benefits for mental and physical health care—for example, establishing lower annual and lifetime limits on mental health care and setting limits on hospital stays for psychiatric needs.

President Bill Clinton released the Health Security Plan in 1993, which was the most comprehensive plan to be proposed at that time since 1965. While that plan did not pass, the Health Insurance Portability and Accountability Act (HIPAA) signed into law in 1996 established privacy and placed restrictions on how preexisting conditions were treated in group health plans, enabling many people with serious mental illness to gain access to health insurance.

In June 1999, President Bill Clinton and Tipper Gore launched a new national campaign to destigmatize mental illness and hosted the first White House Conference on Mental Health. David Satcher, the US Surgeon General, issued a first-of-its-kind report at the end of that year that dealt with mental health and mental illness. The report underscored significant issues the nation was facing in terms of access to care, including racial and financial barriers. In addition, the report charted a course to move ahead that included ensuring parity in physical and mental health care coverage, placing mental illness treatment in the mainstream of health care services, and ensuring consumers access to mental health services that were respectful, evidence based, and reimbursable.

In 2002, President George W. Bush announced the New Freedom Commission on Mental Health, which issued a challenge to transform the nation's mental health system by focusing on community-based care with the goal of recovery. The recovery movement has early roots in Pinel's moral treatment philosophy and the community-based approach of the social settlement movement. Recovery in this context is not defined as curing a chronic mental health condition but is understood as a process through which an individual discovers the means of coping and a sense of their own agency through changing attitudes, values, feelings, goals, skills, and/or roles. The ultimate goal is to enable people with serious mental illness to access the resources they need to live as independently as possible.

The passage of the Mental Health Parity and Addiction Equity Act in 2008 and ACA in 2010 represent significant and hopeful moments regarding mental health care policy in recent memory. Former US representative Patrick Kennedy led the push to pass the Mental Health Parity and Addiction Equity Act, which legally prevents insurance companies from charging higher out-of-pocket costs, restricting stays in the hospital, and limiting the number of therapy visits in their benefit plans for mental health care. Some analysts suggest that the parity act is not enforced with the intensity that is needed. Recent studies show that people with behavioral health issues are far more likely to see out-of-network clinicians largely because of "ghost networks" created by insurance companies. Mental health professionals are typically paid less for their services than their physical health counterparts. According to the Milliman Research Report, the out-of-pocket costs of inpatient mental health care are about thirteen times the rate of all other inpatient care.[7] As a result, only about half of the eight million children who are diagnosed with depression receive treatment. Only about 20 percent of people with substance abuse and addiction disorders get the treatment that they need.[8] ACA enabled twenty-six states to expand Medicaid, the main provider of mental health services for people with serious mental illness. One limitation of the plan, however, is that it does not provide for housing, one of the most desperate needs.

President Trump included repealing and replacing Obamacare in his campaign promises when he ran for election in 2016. The American Health Care Act, also called Trumpcare, passed the House and nearly passed the Senate in 2017. One of the most important differences in this policy is that it reintroduced the ability for insurance companies to exclude coverage for some preexisting conditions, including alcohol and substance abuse, anorexia and bulimia, and major depressive and bipolar disorders.

Neoliberalism represents more than a major change in the understanding of the state's responsibility to provide for the most vulnerable. Neoliberals argue that social entitlement programs perpetuate a culture of poverty. For example, Matt Bevin, former governor of Kentucky, advocated for the state to require residents with disabilities "to work, volunteer, or prepare for jobs in order to receive Medicaid benefits." Bevin suggested that "people in those positions don't need . . . to be treated with the soft bigotry of low expectations."[9] People in poverty or who live on disability benefits are often accused of lacking the motivation to get a job and of gaming or exploiting the welfare system. Within this context, people with disabilities "are treated as economic burdens, redeemable to the point that social and scientific technologies or charities turn [their] bodies into profitable industries."[10]

Limitations of Disability Benefits

One of the biggest fears for people with serious mental illness is losing the disability income, health care benefits, and prescription drug coverage that are essential to their survival. In order to qualify for Social Security Disability Income (SSDI), one first has to make the case that they have a disability. That case must be reviewed and approved. In 2017, one had to earn less than $1,170 per month to qualify for SSDI. The amount can vary according to the disabling condition. You had to earn less than $735 per month to qualify for Social Security Income (SSI).[11] Earnings amounts also change on an annual basis. Moe Armstrong, a military veteran with schizophrenia, expressed his fears related to employment: "One day, I found out I had earned too much income for my [Social Security] benefits and had to pay back $10,000. . . . You have to be very careful not to cross those lines, because you may lose benefits that your boss won't compensate you for."[12] The extremely low limits placed on earning potential for someone receiving SSDI are even more impactful when considering neoliberal arguments that people ought to take personal responsibility to work their way out of poverty. People receiving SSDI find themselves trapped in a catch-22, caught between never having enough income and the precariousness and vulnerability introduced if one earns too much. For them, there is no clear path out of poverty.

Poverty, Precarity, and Potential for Homelessness or Jail Time

Do you remember the story of Eleanor and Christina? Their account helped me grapple on a more personal level with the connection between mental illness and poverty, unemployment, and the potential for homelessness or jail time. Near the end of their parents' lives, it became clear that Christina's social, psychological, and financial needs extended far beyond their financial resources and social network. Eleanor and Christina's parents had always tried to make things better for Christina by providing housing, financial support, and special educational opportunities. At one point, they even paid off Christina's debts to try to prevent her from having a poor credit rating. They were forced to pay nearly $1,200 a month for almost ten years just to keep Christina on her medications because health insurance companies considered her mental illness diagnosis a preexisting condition. Most of their savings were depleted by the time health care policies changed.

The distance between the two sisters shrank quickly after their parents' deaths, and Christina called on Eleanor for help. Eleanor was faced with the choice and challenge of helping Christina find a sustainable housing situation on her very limited SSDI. In order to make it on her own, Christina applied for a Section 8 housing voucher. She had been eligible for some time but resisted applying because her parents paid for her housing. Christina joined hundreds of people on the waiting list for a Section 8 voucher and discovered that the wait could be up to nine years in her area. Christina had to find housing that would allow for a month-to-month lease while she was on the waiting list so she could transition to Section 8 as quickly as possible.

After being on the waiting list for three years, Christina received a letter with the date of her Section 8 briefing. The sisters attended the meeting together and found that they were tasked with finding a landlord within three months who would accept the rental rate established by their metro housing department, fill out and sign detailed paperwork, allow for an inspection, and make repairs to the apartment if needed. Keep in mind that the rental rate and apartment size are determined by a complex formula related to Christina's SSDI and the cost of utilities as opposed to the fair rental value of an apartment. Therefore, Section 8 housing is not in plentiful supply in most cities.

Eleanor described several weeks when she would go with her sister to different rental agencies to help her fill out forms. All of the rental agencies inquired about employment history, rental history, personal references, and income. Christina held only a high school diploma and had lived in relative social isolation with her parents for about ten years, so there was no record of renting an apartment. She could not offer any recent employment history. She did not have enough friends to count on one hand. Christina's credit rating plummeted within a year after her parents' deaths. Eleanor had to cosign for Christina, even with the Section 8 voucher. As I heard their story, I wondered what would happen if Eleanor had chosen not to or was unable to help her sister.

I have interviewed several siblings of people with serious mental illness. Based on many of the stories I heard, Christina is relatively fortunate. The challenges people with mental illness in our society face are so overwhelming and the mental health system is so difficult to navigate and broken that many families feel unable to carry the burden for someone else over the course of their lifetime. In Christina's case, her network of support had become so limited by the time she was in her forties that if any one of these circumstances changed, she could quickly become homeless and unable to access mental health care or medicines on which she depended. She could even end up in jail.

By 2004, 16 percent of prison and jail inmates, or roughly 320,000 people, were seriously mentally ill. That same year, there were about 100,000 psychiatric beds in public and private hospitals. In other words, three times as many mentally ill people were in jail than in a hospital. The governor of Maine proposed in 2007 that some county jails be transformed into special facilities for people with mental illness. Other states followed suit. The Treatment Advocacy Center recently found that by 2014, "approximately 20 percent of inmates in jails and 15 percent of inmates in state prisons have a serious mental illness. . . . This is 10 times more than the approximately 35,000 individuals with serious mental illness remaining in state hospitals."[13] The three largest psychiatric inpatient facilities in the United States today are county jails in Los Angeles, Chicago, and New York. Some states are renovating state asylums, converting them into jails in order to keep up with the need for beds. Neville, another man whom I interviewed who lives with serious mental illness, said, "At least jail is a free place to live."

Disparities in the Distribution of Allocated Resources for Mental Health Care

Today, the United States has one of the highest mental health budgets for services and supports in the world, at about 17 percent of the total health spending budget. But significant disparities persist regarding the distribution of allocated resources and the resulting access to mental health care. Race, sexual orientation, social class, and location are all factors that affect resource allocation and access to mental health care.

For example, only about one-third of Black people who experience psychological distress are able to access adequate mental health care. The availability of mental health services for Black people is primarily through hospitals, community mental health centers, and local federally qualified health centers. Moreover, there is a paucity of psychiatrists, psychologists, and social workers who identify as racial minorities. In 2015, the APA reported that 86 percent of psychologists are white; only 5 percent are Asian, 5 percent are Hispanic, and 4 percent are Black.[14] White mental health professionals lack the experience and often the training in cultural sensitivity necessary to deal with issues faced by clients representing minority groups. As a result, Blacks, Latinx, and other people of minority racial backgrounds are diagnosed with psychotic disorders at three to four times higher rates than whites.

Spending per capita differs tremendously throughout the United States. For example, in my home state of Kentucky, mental health services and supports are only 3 percent of the state's Medicaid budget. Kentucky spends about $55 per capita on mental health compared to the national average of $119.[15] Serious mental illness has a greater impact on states with more rural areas, where access to treatment is more limited and attitudes toward treatment are burdened by stigma and shame. Rural areas are often mental health program service deserts. The National Advisory Committee on Rural Health and the APA report that "more than half of all counties in the U.S. do not have a single psychologist, psychiatrist, or social worker."[16]

The United States also continues to have the most expensive health care system in the world, but the amount spent still does not support the level of care needed. The American Bar Association asserts, "In the U.S. we cannot enjoy the right to health care. The U.S. does not have a health care system, only a health insurance system."[17] Other organizations such as the UN urge countries to reframe mental health policies "in light of the inherent dignity and equality and inalienable rights of all members of the human family."[18]

Empowering Individuals and Families to Gain Control over Their Own Lives

The Western values of individualism, self-sufficiency, and independence have been merged with Christian concepts of charity and self-sacrifice to create policies, systems, and structures that lead to poverty and often prevent people with disabilities and their families from flourishing. What is needed is a new narrative that offers a richer and more textured view of humanity and social redemption.

Christian thought and practices can nurture loving and supportive communities that empower people with serious mental illness and their families to gain control over their own lives. Julie, the mother of an eight-year-old with intellectual and physical disabilities, put it this way: "I can't imagine doing it without God and a faith community on our side." She has two sons: Aiden, who is eleven years old, and Jordan, who is now eight. Jordan is unable to walk due to the malformation of his brain. They are actively involved in a congregation that intentionally created a children's church to enable all of the kids, including those with special needs, to come together and fully participate in activities as equals. Julie says she will never forget the way her church embraces them all as family:

> We were really struggling for a while. My husband was working at a local jail, and I had to quit my job. Our church just started to send us money in the mail. One of the parishioners brought a box of food. We didn't ask for any of it, and we didn't have to prove to anyone our need. We were not going to say we needed help. But people brought us meals and shared our story with us. It was cool to me to think that

we were on their hearts enough just to show up. I can't imagine our life without this support network.

From a theological perspective, we are all created in the image of God. We must consider what that understanding implies for ensuring that basic material and health needs are satisfied and how the Christian moral imagination can move us beyond charity, self-sacrifice, and the prescription for poverty. When considering more specifically Christian concepts of charity and self-sacrifice, a God who requires this approach to dealing with mental illness within the social conditions I have described is more of a burden giver than a friend, source of empowerment, and advocate. The third part of the book will explore biblical threads of empowerment, lift up people and communities that live into a different moral imagination, and suggest an agenda for change.

Empowerment, Alternatives, and Advocacy

CHAPTER FIVE

Biblical Threads of Empowerment

Jesus was teaching in one of the synagogues on the Sabbath. A woman was there who had been disabled by a spirit for eighteen years. She was bent over and couldn't stand up straight. When he saw her, Jesus called her to him and said, "Woman, you are set free from your sickness." He placed his hands on her and she straightened up at once and praised God.

—Luke 13:10–13

Before the advent of disability studies, scant attention was given to examining and writing histories through the lens of people with mental illness and those with other conditions considered disabling. However, this is changing largely due to the impact of scholars such as Brenda Jo Brueggemann, Jay Timothy Dolmage, Paul Longmore, Martha Rose, Susan Sontag, Henri-Jacques Stiker, and Rosemarie Garland Thomson, among others. These scholars raise critical questions about the way we conceive of and represent bodily particularities as we read, write, and reflect on our experiences and history. This chapter will invite you to center your reading of the biblical narrative in the perspectives and experiences of people with serious mental illness and the siblings whom I interviewed. Where can we find threads of empowerment in the Bible to restore, reinforce, and weave a strong social fabric of care to surround and support individuals with serious mental illness and their families?

In this chapter, I will discuss the process of disablement within the context of the ancient world and trace a thread of *empowerment* along lines of beliefs, attitudes, and practices that affirm the whole creation in

God's image. The Holy One sweeps over the waters of chaos and continually creates out of the dark of the deep abyss. Human beings are valued not because of some perceived ideal physical state but because we are created in God's image and increase community. Within the empowerment thread, God partners with the whole creation to bring meaning from the chaos of the human experience and to liberate the human condition. Jesus and Paul confront physiognomy and work with others to transform social hierarchies that privilege the few at the expense of the many.

Constructing Disability in the Greco-Roman World

Early Christian theological interpretations of madness and mania emerged in the context of the ancient Greco-Roman world. Historian Robert Garland says that it is difficult to generalize regarding Roman and Greek attitudes toward deformity and people with disabilities because ideals of beauty and normal morphology are shaped within specific social, cultural, and religious contexts. However, my intention in outlining with broad strokes Roman and Greek views of the body and people with mental and physical impairments is to set the stage for exploring Gospel texts and other early Christian writings regarding healing and demon possessions.

Garland points out that the Greco-Roman world did not "bequeath a serviceable definition for determining what would have been identified as either a deformity or disability."[1] No term directly translated as "disabled" or "disability" exists in the biblical languages of Hebrew and Greek or in church Latin. The Hebrew word *mum* can be translated as "blemish." The Latin word *prodigia*, meaning "wonders" or "miracles," and the Greek term *terata*, meaning "monster," were used more generally in ancient Roman and Greek cultures to refer to people with what Western cultures today identify as disabling or disfiguring conditions.

Unpacking the Power Structures and Constructing Disability in the Ancient World

In order to understand Greek and Roman views of the body—what was considered "disabled" or "deformed"—we need to set them in the context of broader social dynamics, attitudes, and religious beliefs. Ancient Greek and Roman attitudes toward and practices in relation to social difference and vulnerable populations emerge from the prevailing philosophy and religion at the time. A key to understanding the stigmatization of certain populations in antiquity is found by unpacking the power structures.

Balance, Harmony, and Order in Greek and Roman Culture

Greek philosophers valued balance, harmony, and order in nature and society. In the Roman world, the values of the social elite were believed to best reflect order and the status quo and were established by the male householder, or paterfamilias. One's worth was largely social and defined in terms of the good that one contributed to both household and polis. Rosemarie Garland Thomson, humanities scholar and activist for disability justice, suggests that in the "ancient world, the question of 'normalcy' was central. . . . The exclusion and isolation of different bodies were ways to 'reaffirm the unity' of the hegemonic group."[2] The concept of a physical difference or mental illness as a disabling and inferior social position is connected with other factors, including gender, race, social class, citizenship, and ethnicity.

Shaping the Most Beautiful and Ideal Body

The distinction we make between male and female bodies did not exist in the same way in the ancient world. Bodies were understood in terms of a one-sex model. The strong, muscular male body represented the ultimate ideal, and the weaker, fleshier bodies of women and people with mental illness or physical or facial deformities were at the other end of the spectrum. Aristotle thought "All living creatures are dwarf-like compared with man." This belief proceeded "from a reading of the phenomenal world which viewed the human male as the absolute standard of perfection in comparison with which all other animal life is at best deviant, at worst monstrous."[3]

Additionally, ancient Mediterranean constructions of the relationship between the mind and body differed from those that emerged in modernity. French philosopher and historian Michel Foucault thought that before René Descartes, madness was not understood as a turn against the unity of the body, mind, and soul. Premodern thinkers and writers made no categorical distinctions between mind and body. Hippocratic writers, for example, presented mental affections as being of a physical nature and having a physical cause.

The Absence of the Experiences of People with Disabilities in Ancient Histories

There is a lack of clear testimonies that give voice to the lived experiences of ancient people with disabilities. Historians have long assumed that people with disabling conditions and mental illness experienced isolation and were sometimes expelled from their homes and communities. Garland argues they were stigmatized as second-class citizens. Athens was the only city in ancient Greece to create some sort of social entitlement for people living in poverty, many of whom had disabilities. Those suffering from mental ailments appeared to be the worst off in ancient societies. The "feeble-minded and mentally deranged" were barred from holding public office, even when among the elite. Prejudicial social attitudes toward people with disabilities curtailed their political rights, though "whether they were also treated as persons of diminished responsibility in the eyes of the law was unclear."[4]

It is important to note that there is disagreement among historians on this point. Garland has also been challenged for writing an ableist history. Martha Rose applies a disability studies lens to investigate views of physical impairments in *The Staff of Oedipus: Transforming Disability in Ancient Greece*. She limits her study to physical disabilities, but her approach and findings remain relevant to the circumstances of ancient people characterized as mad or demon possessed. Ancient Greeks would not understand the way we view disability in our contemporary society through a primarily medical lens. Rose asserts that people with disabling conditions were not automatically "banned . . . from carrying out certain roles or . . . compartmentalized into others." She argues, "This is not to suggest that the Greeks did not notice physical disability or that physical disability did not have consequences. Rather, the consequences varied from one individual to the next and from one situation to the next."[5] Additionally, positive representations of people with physical impairments come through in Greek literature, such as the character Demosthenes, who overcomes a stutter to become a great orator.[6]

Disability as a Representation of Disorder

Images of physical deformity or people living in poverty were used to represent disorder within the polis and to underscore the contrast to the "well-ordered" behaviors of wealthy people. For example, it became fashionable throughout the Roman Empire for the wealthy to display "human curiosities" in their homes. Hunchbacks, dwarves, and obese women were highly sought after to employ as singers and entertainers.

Social deviance was often ascribed to physical marks, which signified much more than individual moral failures. During economic downturns and times of social unrest, it was easy to cast people considered mad or demon possessed or with physical deformities and foreigners and ethnic minorities along with other marginal groups as menaces or curses to society and to make them scapegoats for social problems. The ancient pseudoscience of physiognomy was used to explain how physical traits revealed an individual's moral character.[7]

Extensive literature references physiognomy in antiquity and the Middle Ages. Aristotle authored the earliest systematic treatise on the subject, which included chapters relating physical characteristics to moral character, strength and weakness, intelligence and stupidity, and so on. Aristotle wrote, "When men have large foreheads, they are slow to move; when they have small ones, they are fickle; when they have broad ones, they are apt to be distraught; when they have foreheads rounded or bulging out they are quick tempered."[8] Other works by the Latin classical writers Juvenal,

Suetonius, and Pliny the Elder as well as Christian authors such as Clement of Alexandria and Origen reference physiognomy. Evidence of the ancient familiarity with physiognomy is found in the Gospel narratives in passages such as Matthew 6:22–23: "The eye is the lamp of the body. Therefore, if your eye is healthy, your whole body will be full of light. But if your eye is bad, your whole body will be full of darkness. If then the light in you is darkness, how terrible that darkness will be!"

Connecting Wealth and Poverty to Disability

Poverty was rife in ancient Greece and Rome. Wealthy people showed some concern for philanthropy and sharing, but their benevolence was "primarily toward one's own people, parents, and other family members, and guests or to strangers, not toward the poor." They identified joy with giving, but their motivation resided in the pursuit of "honour, prestige, fame, status."[9]

The gods were believed to be on the side of the wealthy rather than the impoverished majority. Pieter van der Horst, a scholar of early Christian literature, writes, "There was a Zeus *Xenios* (for strangers) and a Zeus *Hiketêsios* (for supplicants), but there was no Zeus *Ptôchios* (for the poor), nor any other god with an epithet indicating concern for the needy. It was rather the rich who were seen as the favourites of the divine world, their wealth being the visible proof of that favour."[10] It was a commonly held belief that the wealthy were morally superior to the people living in poverty.

Wealthy people could distance themselves from people living in poverty and relied on the labor of other bodies to display their status and to navigate their own physical impairments. The term *stigma* originated within this context to identify physical marks that branded slaves and criminals so that their place within the social strata would be easily discernable. Those with the financial means to do so owned slaves. In ancient cities, slaves transported the wealthiest on litters (*lecticae*) and sedan chairs (*sellae*).[11] Moreover, slavery could be the cause of disabling conditions because masters commanded slaves to do risky work to minimize their own vulnerabilities. Poverty itself could also lead to disability; poor sanitation and nutrition were among other causes of blindness and deafness.

Tracing the Empowerment Thread

Jesus and his early followers lived primarily as the impoverished majority in the Roman Empire and resisted and rejected the motto of classical humanism, which was to give to those who the social elites considered deserving. The Torah was central to Jesus's religious observance of God's commandments. Among Jewish people, the concept of *tzedakah*, meaning "righteousness in the sense of justice," revealed something about the nature of God and reflected commandments to care for people in poverty and to honor the whole creation as God's own.

Followers of Jesus advocated for the redistribution of wealth among the most marginalized and vulnerable and thus defined themselves as a countercultural movement.[12] For example, Jesus preached the Sermon on the Mount (Matthew 5:3–11) to large crowds of people who were hungry—literally famished. As he claimed the expansiveness of God's blessing for the poor in spirit, the meek, those who mourn, the merciful, and those who suffer for the sake of righteousness, he challenged the preferred ordering of the household in the Roman Empire. Margaret Aymer, a scholar of Christian scriptures, translates the Greek term *makarioi* used in this passage as "greatly honored" rather than "blessed" in order to emphasize the way Jesus understood God in the midst of life-provisioning activities.[13]

Knowing the Torah Well

In Hebrew, the first book of the Torah bears a different name than Genesis—*bereshit*, or "beginnings," especially as it relates to the activity of creation. Gregory Mobley, a professor of Hebrew Bible and congregational studies at Yale Divinity School, suggests that the ancient authors of the Hebrew Scriptures grappled with one primary theme: God's partnership with the whole creation to bring meaning from the chaos of experience in order to liberate the human condition.[14] Liberating the human condition involves expanding care in community through hospitality, particularly for those living in the most vulnerable circumstances—the stranger, the alien, the widow, and other people in poverty.

Paying Attention to the Backstory

We are often prone to read Genesis 1 as establishing an order for creation, but understanding the cosmology of the Hebrew Bible—or the backstory, as Mobley calls it—suggests that the story invites us to think more about the rhythm of God's continual creativity than a single event. Another Near Eastern creation story, the *Enuma Elish*, informed the theological and social imaginary of Genesis 1. The *Enuma Elish* is a Mesopotamian creation myth about a storm god and patron of Babylon named Marduk, who is in a desperate battle to defeat chaos. Marduk overcomes Mother Ocean in primordial times. Then he uses the parts of her body to give order to the world and contends with another goddess named Tiamat, depicted as a sea dragon, and her eleven chaos monsters. When Marduk defeats Tiamat, he uses her body parts to continue to create the world. One of the things about great storytelling is that you can never keep the monsters that create chaos completely down; they always return. Symbolically, "the chaos monsters are personifications of the disorderly, random, and untamed features of reality. The backstory explains that God has defeated but not obliterated the monsters, and that they invariably return to wreak havoc when humans inadvertently open the door to their cages through ethical lapses."[15]

Tiamat's shadow looms in the minds of the writers of Genesis and "appears, not as a personified serpent, but as instead *tehom*, its Hebrew cognate meaning 'the abyss.'" Within the creation story, *ruach elohim*, the "breath of God," hovers over the abyss to produce life-sustaining patterns for the whole creation out of chaos. Throughout Genesis 1, the writers include a refrain—"God saw how good it was" (see Genesis 1:10)—which reinforces, reminds, and instructs us of continual divine creative activity. Humans bring back the monsters of chaos in story after story, and God consistently sends forth the breath that animates life, restores harmony, rebuilds cities and relationships in ruin, and creates life-sustaining communities of belonging out of devastation, chaos, exile, and isolation.

For example, think about the story of Moses. Moses is born during a time of tremendous crisis, when the ancient Hebrew people are living in slavery in Egypt and threatened by the deadly policies of the Egyptian leader (see Exodus 2). When Moses was born, his mother hid him for three months. In the chaos of her time, she is forced to set him adrift in a waterproof basket to protect him from Pharaoh's orders that midwives murder newborn baby boys. The baby, however, is discovered by a princess, Pharaoh's daughter, when she goes down to bathe in the Nile. She sends her attendants to retrieve the basket from the water and finds a nursemaid for Moses whom the story reveals is his mother, and she secretly nurtures her son. The princess chooses a name for Moses and explains its meaning in Hebrew: "to draw out." Moses's naming represents his experience of living in two cultures. Later, God collaborates and partners with Moses, who leads the Hebrew people on the Exodus journey, parting the Red Sea to cut through the chaos and trauma inflicted by Pharaoh's empire and provide safe passage to the Promised Land. One of the Ten Commandments given to Moses reminds the Hebrew people not to make an idol in the form of heaven above or on the earth beneath or in the waters below because the God of the Exodus journey overcomes the chaos symbolized by the water (see Exodus 20:4–5). This story was passed on to help generations survive exile, violence, and the chaos and trauma inflicted by imperial rule.

The idea of God creating by subduing chaos carries through into prophetic writings and then later into Gospel narratives and Paul's theological reflections. Robert Gnuse, a biblical scholar and professor of humanities at Loyola University New Orleans, says that Second Isaiah merges the imagery of God as creator of the world with that of God as liberator:

> Awake, awake, put on strength,
>   arm of the Lord.
> Awake as in times past,
>   generations long ago.
> Aren't you the one who crushed Rahab,
>   who pierced the dragon?

Didn't you dry up the sea,
      the waters of the great deep?
And didn't you make the redeemed a road to cross
      through the depths of the sea,
      a road for the redeemed to pass? (Isaiah 51:9–10)

The ancient combat imagery of creation in Isaiah 51 suggests that God's parting of the Red Sea for the Israelites to cross during the Exodus journey is reminiscent of Marduk's primordial defeat of the goddess Tiamat by cutting the water in half.

Holiness Codes, "Blemished Bodies," and God's Care

The holiness codes also deepen our understanding of the empowerment thread. Anthropologist Mary Douglas argues that rituals of purity and piety in the ancient world were intended to reorder the social environment to conform to a particular idea of order or moral code.[16] The body protects the demarcation lines between chaos and meaninglessness with that of order and holiness. Leviticus 19:2 introduces the intention or purpose of the holiness codes: "Say to the whole community of the Israelites: You must be holy, because I, the Lord your God, am holy." The Hebrew word translated here as *holy* literally means "set apart." Each injunction calls attention to the way that God works through human affairs and intends to create an order through which the community receives God's blessing.

One passage from the holiness codes that contributed to views of disability in Western societies discusses rules of Levitical priesthood:

The Lord spoke to Moses, saying: Speak to Aaron and say: No one of your offspring throughout their generations who has a blemish may approach to offer the food of his God. For no one who has a blemish shall draw near, one who is blind or lame, or one who has a mutilated face or a limb too long, or one who has a broken foot or a broken hand, or a hunchback, or a dwarf, or a man with a blemish in his eyes or an itching disease or scabs or crushed testicles.... He may eat the food of his God, of the most holy as well as of the holy. But he shall not come near the curtain or approach the altar, because he has a blemish, that he may not profane my sanctuaries; for I am the Lord; I sanctify them. Thus Moses spoke to Aaron and to his sons and to all the people of Israel. (Leviticus 21:16–20, 22–24 NRSV)

Biblical scholar Amos Yong reminds us that passages such as this cannot be taken out of context. Discriminating against or disempowering people with disabilities is not the primary concern of the codes included in Leviticus 21. What it means to be set apart is found in other injunctions in Leviticus: "You must not insult a deaf person or put some obstacle in front of a blind person that would cause them to trip. Instead, fear your God; I am the Lord" (Leviticus 19:14). Yong writes, "People with disabilities are also the special objects of divine care, often in connection with the poor, the oppressed, and the marginalized."[17] People in poverty, those who are oppressed and marginalized, widows, and the stranger are taken more and more into community and act as partners with God throughout the stories told in the Hebrew Bible.

Heroes with Disabling Conditions in the Hebrew Bible

Stories throughout the Hebrew Bible capture a sense of the depth of God's presence and activity throughout creation, which is *b'tzelem elohim*: "Then God said, 'Let us make humanity in our image to resemble us so that they may take charge of the fish of the sea, the birds in the sky, the livestock, all the earth, and all the crawling things on earth.' God created humanity in God's own image" (Genesis 1:26–27). God creates within and among characters living in varied and complex circumstances. What is distinct about these characters is that they respond to and partner with God to provision for life in frequently unjust social conditions.

Characters with physical impairments or mental illness aren't merely objects of charity; they are also the heroes of the story. God doesn't work only through "unblemished" bodies. Stories in the Hebrew Bible reference physical distinctions, but the essence of the characters is never solely defined by their state of impairment. Physical characteristics are also not ancillary to the theological imagination informing biblical stories.

Sometimes a disabling condition is the means for God to reveal Godself. For example, Jacob limps after he wrestles with God (Genesis 32:31). Leah has "delicate" eyes (Genesis 29:17). Miriam has a skin disease, likely leprosy (Numbers 12:10–11). Moses stutters and relies on his brother Aaron to speak for him (Exodus 4:10–16). Saul experiences depression and bouts of insanity (1 Samuel 10:21–23; 11:5–7; 16:14). This idea carries through into the Gospels. Remember that Zechariah, Elizabeth's husband, cannot speak when he refuses to believe that they will have a child (Luke 1:13–25).

Jesus Setting Limits to Chaos

The empowerment thread is evident throughout the Gospels when reading Jesus's story through the eyes of the demon possessed, the unclean, and the paralytic. Consider reading the Gospel of Mark by replacing each reference to the sea and water with the word *chaos* and reflect on the narrative in light of the experience of the demon possessed. John baptizes Jesus. While Jesus "was coming up out of the water, Jesus saw heaven splitting open and the Spirit, like a dove, coming down on him. And there was a voice from heaven: 'You are my Son, whom I dearly love; in you I find happiness'" (Mark 1:10–11). Immediately, Jesus is forced out into the wilderness.

After calling the disciples and traveling with them to Capernaum, Jesus enters a synagogue where he amazes people with his teaching. A person with an evil spirit screams after recognizing that Jesus is "the holy one from God" (Mark 1:24). The disciples in Mark never know who Jesus is; the demon-possessed person consistently recognizes him.

In Mark 4, Jesus miraculously sets limits beyond which the waters of chaos cannot pass. Jesus had just been teaching the disciples and the crowds with parables about the kingdom of God. Later that day, they get into a boat to cross over the sea (chaos). Jesus is in the boat with the disciples, and they wonder how he can sleep. After the disciples wake Jesus up, the narrative reports that "the wind settled down and there was a great calm" (Mark 4:39). The next miraculous act Jesus performs after calming the storm is setting a demon-possessed man—often seen howling in the tombs nearby his hometown—free from his chains and leg irons.

Jesus embodies the most generous aspects of his Jewish tradition as he works within and through the chaos that human beings experience and inflict on each other as they create artificial yet tangible boundaries and then decide who can flourish in or outside the lines. In ancient societies where the body protected the demarcation lines between chaos and meaninglessness and order and holiness, Jesus's miraculous acts heal by challenging the ordering of the household that was intended to uphold and reinforce the power of social elites. Jesus travels the countryside where people exiled from their communities are forced to live, enters into the tombs where people are howling, touches those who have been bleeding for years, and goes to the places where people are crying to awaken a young girl who wouldn't or couldn't wake up. Those possessed by so-called evil spirits recognize him.

Healing as Empowerment

In the Gospel of Mark alone, nearly one-third of the narrative concerns itself with Jesus's miraculous acts, including healing stories about people who experience blindness, deafness, paralysis, leprosy, and demon possession. These tales respond directly to the preferred ordering of the household of the Roman Empire and clarify the teachings of Jesus's Jewish tradition by claiming the expansiveness of God's blessing. Jesus does not view "blemished" bodies simply as ancillary to the lives of social elites or valued according to what they contribute to individual households or mark them as slaves.

In the story of the bent-over woman (Luke 13:10–17), Luke underscores the woman's condition by describing her as someone disabled by a spirit—bent over and unable to stand up straight. Biblical scholar Gregory Lamb observes, "Such a vivid description echoes ancient physiognomic assumptions regarding those having twisted or crooked backs."[18] Strong backs were associated with good moral character, weak backs with feeble character. But Jesus draws near to the woman. He places his hands on her, which challenges the social distance ancient society required of men and women, powerful and powerless. He says, "Woman, you are set free." She stands up for herself. In Jesus's act of empowerment, he proclaims a radical vision of social transformation and solidarity where people are valued because of their creation in God's image and welcomed as agents of change.

Paul's Empowerment as the First Theologian with a Disability

The empowerment thread is also evident in Paul's letters as he writes to newly forming communities of faith throughout the Roman Empire. Theologian Amos Yong suggests that Paul is likely one of the first theologians to write out of his own experience of living with a disability. In 2 Corinthians, Paul describes living with a thorn—in Greek, *skolops*. Second Corinthians 12:7 is the only place that *skolops* appears in the Christian Scriptures.[19] Many theories seek to explain the thorn Paul describes. The text indicates that Paul had eye trouble, something that disfigured his face and made him hard to look at. Others think he had epilepsy. Emotional trauma is also a plausible interpretation of the thorn in Paul's flesh. Biblical scholars agree that Paul wrestled with a great deal of hardship. Whatever the ailment was, it bothered him immensely, and he prayed earnestly for God to rid him of it.

I don't think it is of great consequence to our interpretation of Paul's experience of the thorn to understand the specific nature of his ailment. It is far more significant to consider what his physical differences represented in an ancient culture that valued physiognomy. Within that context, Paul's experiences empowered him to challenge those who held the power and privilege to determine and identify beauty and good moral character.

The superapostles, Paul's opponents, use the invective of physiognomy against him. They hone in on his perceived physical limitations to underscore the threat of his speech: "I know what some people are saying: 'His letters are severe and powerful, but in person he is weak and his speech is worth nothing'" (2 Corinthians 10:10).[20] This attitude betrays a whole range of prejudices through which the superapostles judge how people size up to Rome's elite, who set the bar for the ideal. In the face of these insults, Paul questions why he has to be the one to have this thorn in the flesh. He realizes through more reflection that there is something much larger at stake. Paul wrestles with his own thorn and concludes that the good news for his time is that God claims him as made in God's image within a society that builds itself up by exclusion—exclusion of the different, the dwarf, the hunchback, the woman, and the slave, all those whose identities were reduced to traits considered undesirable and undeserving.

What Does It Mean for Jesus and Paul to Be Demon Possessed?

You may find it intriguing that *foolishness*, *madness*, *demon*, and *demon possession* are terms used in Christian Scriptures to single out Paul and Jesus because of the ways they challenge the power structures supporting the social hierarchy of their day. Soon after Jesus announces his public ministry in Mark, Matthew, and Luke, he begins to throw out or expel evil spirits and demons and heal a range of diseases. Various symptoms are named to represent demon possession throughout the Gospels; some can be identified as deformity and specific ailments such as epilepsy. Ultimately, it is Jesus who receives the strongest accusation of demon possession because he refuses to uphold the status quo: "The legal experts came down from Jerusalem. Over and over they charged, 'He's possessed by Beelzebul. He throws out demons with the authority of the ruler of demons'" (Mark 3:22).

Paul employs the terms *madness* or *foolishness* in defense of his commitment to the Gospel throughout 1 and 2 Corinthians. In 2 Corinthians 11, he defends himself against the charges made by the superapostles by asking the faith community at Corinth to bear with his madness. He applies the language of weakness in a similar fashion as the medical writers of the time. On one level, Paul uses madness and weakness to align himself with Christ. On another level, Paul does not completely subvert the meaning of weak bodies and mental capacity. He makes an effort to uphold norms of masculinity when he boasts about his own authority. But when he speaks of his leadership of different communities, he uses feminine language. New Testament scholar Beverly Gaventa traces Paul's use of maternal imagery in her book *Our Mother St. Paul.*[21] She asserts that Paul draws on maternal imagery to refer to his nurturing of and ongoing relationship with different congregations. This too would have been a challenge to the ancient status quo. Paul's response to his adversaries was to identify with the weakest. He claims on numerous occasions in his letter that Christ's power rests in his weakness. These statements directly challenge and resist the dominant hierarchical scale on which people in his culture measured different bodies.

Recalling the Stories of Siblings

In the previous chapter, I shared some of the ways that siblings reflect theologically on their own experiences. I lifted up examples of siblings who had difficulty grappling with questions related to the meaning and purpose of disabilities and needed new ways of speaking about God's presence in the midst of their experience of family life. Recall the way that Adair reflected on her experience of Christian community and the "God she needed" after her brother's suicide: "What I needed was a God who can do triage every day." Glenn also spoke about how God empowers him in his role as a caregiver: "God is a gracious God and not a stern restrictive God but an expansive God. God includes all people, even my brother. My hope for my brother and my family is that we would experience God in the midst of community like that."

The empowerment thread as described here invites a very different way of thinking about God's active presence in the lives of families affected by serious mental illness. Jesus sets limits to the chaos we experience in our lives, calms storms, and embodies a radical social transformation as he confronts physiognomy. Through acts of self-giving love and solidarity, Christ empowers partnership in community and provides hope, meaning, and purpose. People with mental and physical impairments are not just objects of charity; they act as agents of change and reveal divine activity. In the next chapter, I will provide several examples of individuals and communities that weave the empowerment thread into their daily routines, nurture self-giving love, create belonging, and provision for the well-being of all, particularly families affected by serious mental illness.

CHAPTER SIX

Communities of Empowerment and Belonging

No matter what, don't give anyone crazy looks. Don't judge anyone. Just say you will be there for them and be there for them. Bring the community together and actually help this person. . . . Use the community to back this person up and whoever has the mental illness to help them. Be there for them. I guess that is all I would say.

—Jade

I shared some of Dorothy's interview in a previous chapter. Dorothy is the primary caregiver for her younger brother Peter who has schizoaffective disorder bipolar type. She and Peter live in a very supportive and empowering community. Their home is near a college campus that she described as a "kind of village." Dorothy said, "Community helps make my care of Peter possible and my ability not to be stopped by other things because of that responsibility." People who live in the village watch out for each other. When Dorothy travels for work, neighbors check in on Peter. She observed, "At our best, we ought to just know that people are going to be there to support our family, especially the most vulnerable members of our community, and it is hard sometimes. My brother is not the most communicative person. But even the kids in this village get it. Once you know what to expect, people get used to it, and they just kind of get it and invite you in in interesting ways."

Grace reflected on how her brother Will transformed her view of God and community:

What has it done to my faith? It has made it exponentially stronger because you can't afford shallow faith. So we can never take for granted anything, especially in my home. . . . We have to love and embrace our siblings and other people with mental illness because we do not define their worth. Their worth is in their creation in the image of God. That is the call to people like me, as a Christian and as a sibling. When there was not rational reason, I had to tap into what is not default human behavior and appeal to that function that is more in the likeness of God. I can love you because you are part of the substance of what makes us all human. That is what the Christian community is called to do.

This chapter is all about Christian communities called to "function more in the likeness God," as Grace describes. To find these stories, I have looked for people and communities that pick up the empowerment thread and create alternatives within the context of their time to the primary approaches to caregiving and treatment of serious mental illness. The stories of Hildegard of Bingen and Sigewize; Dietrich Bonhoeffer and his experience at Bethel; the foster community in Geel, Belgium; the L'Arche communities; and the ministries of Dismas Charities—the Diersen House illustrate just a few communities of care that emphasize mutuality, reciprocity, and self-giving love.

Hildegard and Human Beings as the Microcosm of Creation

Some of Hildegard of Bingen's story will seem fantastic and strange to readers in the twenty-first century. But within the context of her time, Hildegard's integrated approach to healing stands out as distinct. She was a mystic, philosopher, musician, medical practitioner, and religious woman who earned a reputation for recognizing the complexity of human identities and embracing people as "microcosms of creation."[1]

In 1169, an abbot named Gedolphus wrote to Hildegard to seek her advice about how to care for Sigewize, a noblewoman of Brauweiler.

Sigewize had been besieged by a "demon" for seven years. Hildegard was well known for her medical knowledge and ability to heal. In her reply to Abbot Gedolphus, Hildegard included clear written directions for priests to perform an exorcism. She instructed seven priests each who would play the role of a biblical character during the ceremony to "strike Sigewize lightly with rods on her head, back, navel, knees and feet, while chanting 'Now you, O satanic and evil spirit, you who oppress and torment this person, this form of a woman, depart.'" After the chant, the priests were to offer several more blows and demand the spirit to leave. The priests carried out the exorcism, but it proved effective only for a brief time. Exorcism in the Middle Ages was seen as a way to continue Jesus's acts of healing as described in Gospel passages such as Mark 5:1–9, where an unclean spirit is cast out of the man living in the tombs. Some believed that a demon could entrap or imprison a person's soul.[2] When the exorcism failed, Sigewize was sent to Hildegard and the nuns at the cloistered community of Rupertsberg, where they took a more integrated approach to her healing.

Monastic communities served as repositories for medical knowledge well into the twelfth century. Hildegard had access to substantial libraries and gained medical knowledge from the many visitors to her cloistered community. Historians today remain fascinated by Hildegard's integrative approach to medical arts, as she did not establish clear boundaries among the medical, magical, and miraculous ways of healing.

In *Causae et Curae*, Hildegard described her understanding of human nature and the causes of melancholy and madness. Human beings were part of a much larger story as a "microcosm of creation." According to Hildegard, physical and mental problems were first introduced into human history at the point of Adam's disobedience. Black bile originated from Adam's semen through the breath of the serpent at the fall. Depression resulted from many factors related to mood, actions and choices, the humors, the moistness and dryness and sweetness of the body and the brain, the afterlife, and the elements. She writes that when dry and moist humors exceed "their proper amount, like a wave in the water that becomes too big, they change themselves into poison. A tempest arises out of them in such a way that no humor can be balanced with any other and they no longer carry out their task.... Any person who suffers this opposition and contradiction in his body will become mad."[3] Of course, you will recognize some ways that Hildegard's story reflects the beliefs and practices of her time. But her approach is of greater interest to us because she offers an example of someone in the Middle Ages who made a significant departure from the dominant attitudes and approaches to caregiving and the treatment of people considered to be demon possessed.

When Sigewize arrived at the cloister, Hildegard paid special attention to her diet, made sure she was included in all daily routines of the religious community, and attended to the spiritual dimension of her illness. Sigewize lived as a novice at Rupertsberg until her death. Because of their gender, women mystics always had to be conscious of the tightrope they were walking between their own intuitive experience of God and what others may think of as madness. Maybe this consciousness gave Hildegard some special insight into what Sigewize was experiencing.

Dietrich Bonhoeffer's Social Christology and the Responsibility to Care for Each Other

The writings and actions of Lutheran theologian Dietrich Bonhoeffer provide an example from a different era of the ways Christian communities live in the likeness and image of God. Bonhoeffer challenged flawed concepts of "well-born" superhumans and proclaimed the responsibility of church and society to live in self-giving love and to provision for the well-being of all. Two experiences played key roles in shaping Bonhoeffer's Christology and our responsibility to care for each other: visits to Harlem during a year that he studied at Union Theological Seminary in New York and time spent at Bethel, a community of care for people with disabilities in Bielefeld, Germany.

Ethicist Reggie Williams observes that Bonhoeffer argued for a social Christology that responded to the neurotic Nazi obsession with human perfection, "good" genes, being "well-born," and ordered life. Bonhoeffer was studying at Union Theological Seminary during the same year that

Thomas Shipp and Abraham Smith were lynched in the town center of Marion, Indiana. Photos of the bodies of two Black men hanging from the trees while townspeople stood around glaring at the spectacle as if they were viewing a freak show became the inspiration for the song "Strange Fruit," which was written by Abel Meeropol and popularized by blues singer Billie Holiday. News of the event spread worldwide as it was captured by Holiday's hauntingly beautiful voice. Reading the poetry of the Harlem Renaissance and witnessing firsthand Black suffering throughout his travels in the United States, including in the Jim Crow South, clarified the meaning of Jesus's actions for Bonhoeffer.

The story of Jesus could only be understood by firmly placing it within his historical context. Bonhoeffer thought that distorted images of Christ made in the likeness of the white power brokers of Western societies taught Christians to ignore the daily conditions of human existence or to protect their own social status. He articulated the concept of *Stellvertretung*, which means roughly "God taking our place," to open up the possibility of a Christ who lives in the experiences of slaves, outcasts, and the marginalized and who enters into the crawl spaces of people's lives in self-giving love. God reveals Godself "not in the glory of human aptitude for all to see, but in hiddenness, through suffering, and shame."[4]

In 1933, not too long after Bonhoeffer returned to Europe from New York, he was asked to go on retreat with other religious leaders at Bethel, a settlement for the care of people with epilepsy and disabilities. The Lutheran Church started a seminary there so that pastors could be trained at the same time they lived and ministered among those experiencing a variety of illnesses. Bonhoeffer shared in a letter to his grandmother his experience of what church looked like at Bethel:

> Here we have a part of the church that still knows what the church can be about and what it cannot be about. I have just come back from the worship service. It is an extraordinary sight, the whole church filled with crowds of epileptics and other ill persons, interspersed with the deaconesses and deacons who are there to help in case one of them falls; then there are elderly tramps who come in off the country roads, the theological students, the children from the lab school, doctors

and pastors with their families. But the sick people dominate the picture, and they are keen listeners and participants. . . . There is nothing sentimental about any of this; it is tremendously real and natural. It knocks down some of the barriers with which we usually shut ourselves off from this world.[5]

The occasion for his retreat at Bethel was to work with other church leaders on a confessional statement to confront German Christians supporting the Nazis and to clarify the mission and prophetic voice of the church during the height of the eugenics movement and a time of tremendous polarization. Eugenics was not only being promoted in Germany at that time, and Bonhoeffer would have been aware of the growth of sterilization laws in the United States. Forty-eight US states had passed laws to prevent certain groups of people from perpetuating "bad genes" by the time the church leaders began working on their statement in 1933. The first draft of the Bethel Confession reformulated Christian doctrines in response to faulty and reductive interpretations made by the German Christians and challenged their interpretation of the cross promoted in the Nazi slogan, "Public interest before self-interest," and their emphasis on the "law of race." Central to the confession was the idea that all people are created in the image of God and therefore have a value and inherent right beyond one's social usefulness.

Bernd Wannenwetsch observes that the community at Bethel provided Bonhoeffer and other church leaders with the view they needed from below to clearly expose the anti-Christian nature of the Aryan superhuman in contrast to embodied Christian anthropology.[6] A community of belonging cannot be identified with the "worship of power." For Bonhoeffer, Christians must also avoid the perilous middle ground of taking up the common charitable attitude toward the weak if it meant that they maintained their own position of social authority and power. He proclaimed in a sermon on Paul's concept of power in weakness, "Whenever a man is in physical or social or moral or religious weakness is aware of his existence and likeness with God, there he is sharing in God's life, there he feels God being with him, there he is open for God's life, there he is open for God's strength, that is God's grace, God's love, God's comfort, which passeth all understanding and all human values."[7] The role of the church within this context was to be the real material form of Christ's existence in the world, an existence that embodied authentic humanity in love, not perfection. Bonhoeffer's writings and experiences suggest to us that caring for each other is a responsibility that extends far beyond ties of biological kinship to a much larger community.

Geel and the Strange Healing Powers of Not Trying to Fix the Problem

The convents of Rupertsberg and Bethel are not the only examples of communities of care that existed in the Western European context and aimed to empower all of their members and embody belonging. Geel, Belgium, is the place where Dymphna, the patron saint of people with mental illness, is believed to have been martyred. Legend holds that five "lunatics" spent the night in the place where she was killed and were healed. In the fourteenth century, a church was built on top of her remains. That church became a pilgrimage site for people struggling with mental health issues, and for centuries, villagers welcomed the pilgrims to stay in their homes.

Today, the villagers of Geel continue that practice through a sort of fostering program. *Invisibilia*, a podcast of National Public Radio, covered the story of Geel and discusses their approach to caregiving. People with mental illness there are never called *patients*, but always *boarders* or *guests*. When the guests arrive, they do receive some psychiatric treatment and necessary prescriptions and are assigned a therapist, but hosts never label them with a diagnosis. Several people interviewed in Geel suggested that the psychiatric profession focusing on recovery and the medical model can cloud one's ability to see people as they really are.

At the heart of Geel's approach is the idea that people with mental illness are "a part of normal life."[8] A villager named Gaston Van Dyke said, "The philosophy behind that is first, you have to accept mentally ill people. You have to accept what they are doing." Accepting the fact that you don't have to make odd behaviors like hallucinations, constant motion, or blurting things out go away redefines the norms of the community.

Geel distinguishes itself by not looking at people as problems to be fixed or simply as objects of care; instead, it focuses on working around and with the guests' peculiarities. Caregivers and boarders affirm each other's humanity and accept one another as they are.

Christian Friendship and the L'Arche Community

Jason Greig, a theologian in the Mennonite tradition, brings to light more "practices, values, and narratives a community must have to faithfully assist everyone to grow into their vocation as truly human persons."[9] Greig begins his book on *Reconsidering Intellectual Disability* with Ashley's story. Ashley is a young woman born with what doctors defined as profound intellectual and physical disabilities. She will be completely reliant on her parents for her physical care, and like so many other families whose stories are told in these pages, they will shoulder the burden of caring for their daughter for her entire lifetime. Due to the weight of the burden of care, doctors and the medical ethics board at the hospital recommended that her parents choose to limit Ashley's physical growth by removing her breast buds and uterus so that she would always be small and childlike and thus easier to care for. "The Ashley Treatment" is now used as a case study for debates in medical ethics. Ashley's treatment highlights the social context in which families are forced to make desperate decisions due to the oppressive weight of family burden and how people with disabilities are treated as objects of care.

Greig considers Ashley's extreme treatment the result of the late modern social imaginary that defines relationships primarily by mutual consent and equality of symmetrical ability. "For the self of Western liberation," Greig writes, "legitimate moral discourse must be self-determining and self-originating."[10] The medical model within this framework reduces people with disabilities to "defective bodies" and treats them almost solely as objects of care. Those who lack the capacity for self-representation are disqualified from moral discourse and from intimate relationships of friendship and mutuality.

In contrast, Greig observes that the Christian social imaginary begins with the assumption that interdependence is our state of being and the creation itself has a value beyond social utility. For Greig, the Trinity is the central Christian symbol that expresses God's life of interdependence and models love and self-giving in relationship. Christians know life as beings created by a good God; we apprehend that human limitations manifest a more truthful description of reality and embrace our bodies as they truly are.

One of the Christian practices that Greig emphasizes is foot washing because it honors our embodied realities. Jesus washes the disciples' feet and, by doing so, "shows the mutuality of his relationship with them, and gives them an example of the character that their ensuing relationships in the ecclesia must embody. The relationships in the Body of Christ must be marked by the mutual hospitality and receptivity."[11]

Greig underscores the importance of the L'Arche communities as an expression of Christian friendship. Jean Vanier started the first community of L'Arche so that men and women with disabling conditions could share their lives together along with others called to live with them. In order to deal with Vanier's writings with integrity, I think it is important to introduce his work with an awareness that the L'Arche community discovered and confirmed that Vanier harassed and engaged in manipulative sexual relationships with women from 1970 to 2005. My intention here is not to lift Vanier up as a morally exemplary individual but rather to emphasize how L'Arche communities interpret and embody aspects of his thinking.

For Vanier, there was no particular theoretical launch point to begin L'Arche. His primary aim was to be "open to providence and daily life" and to discern what belonging to each other and living together reveals about God in the midst of daily life. The story of Jesus is intended not to recommend a particular moral position or feeling we should have about those who are victimized by society but rather to raise questions about who truly is our neighbor. In *Befriending the Stranger*, Vanier writes,

> There is much inside of us that we do not want to look at.
> People with alcohol problems, for example, rarely recognize or
>   admit that they are addicted.
> Jesus wants to teach us to know ourselves
>   with our gifts, with our beauty,

with our deepest desire to love,
with our pain, our fragility, our vulnerability.[12]

It is worth speculating on the profoundness of Vanier's reflections in light of his work with L'Arche and his own inability to be honest about his sexual abuse. His own brokenness and the pain he inflicted on others may have introduced him to a deeper understanding of the depth of love and hospitality to the stranger one needs in Christ.

Making Connections between Empowerment and Provisioning for Life in Community

The stories of the people and communities told in this chapter invite us to think about how the empowerment of individuals and families affected by serious mental illness is so deeply connected to affirming humans as "microcosms of creation," provisioning for the variability of conditions we experience throughout our lives, and love embodied in relationship. The empowering and life-provisioning actions of another community caught me by surprise when I visited Dismas Charities–Diersen (Diersen House). Diersen House is a halfway house for women who are either currently incarcerated or have been recently paroled subject to being released upon the completion of a six-month substance abuse program. Women are assigned there in different ways. All are struggling with substance abuse issues. Many have co-occurring conditions related to mental illness. Like many other states, good-quality mental health care is in short supply in Kentucky; the state ranks fortieth in the United States for access to care by primary physicians. Only about half of the adults who struggle with mental health issues get the care they need, which also impacts substance abuse and suicide rates.

New Life in Christ Christian Church meets in Diersen House weekly and brings together people from outside churches to worship with the women living there. Anyone can be a member of New Life; you don't have to be "doing time" at Diersen. New Life also works in collaboration with other local congregations to plan and host worship. I work with the pastor on different occasions on community engagement opportunities at Diersen for students taking my classes. There, the college students learn to build and navigate relationships across many socially constructed boundaries used to define differences among us as human beings—gender, age, sexual orientation, race, class, economic condition, mental and physical ability and impairment, and so on. Diersen House is an excellent context for these experiences because it affords some freedom to the women living there even as a lockdown facility and enables mutual exchange.

Women living at Diersen wear street clothes but cannot leave the facility except in supervised group outings. They must check in at particular times, complete chores assigned to them, and participate in meetings and other planned sessions. Members of the local community who are visitors of New Life have to be buzzed in and then sign a roster in order to participate in worship and other events. A staff member of the Diersen House facility sitting behind a large double-paned glass panel monitors the whole process.

The facility is a former elementary school, and the worshipping community usually convenes in a multipurpose room set up cafeteria-style, with long tables that each seat about twenty people. All people gathering for worship can choose their own seats. Worship blends a variety of Christian traditions and incorporates a lot of singing. Local churches also volunteer to plan and lead the service so the responsibility doesn't rest solely on the New Life pastor or the women housed at Diersen. The order of worship is often creative and includes some elements specifically related to the context, like the call-and-response introduction of each worship leader in the style of Alcoholics Anonymous that is threaded throughout the service.

This particular visit occurred during the week before Easter Sunday and incorporated another special element in the service on that Tuesday evening, the ritual of foot washing. Near the end of the service, everyone who wants to have their feet washed is invited by two worship leaders to go forward to two washing stations set up in the aisle between the tables. You could then sit down in a chair, and the worship leader for that washing station would help you take off your shoes and gently wash your feet and then dry them with a towel. Inspirational music started playing, and a few people began to walk forward. As you can imagine, not everyone dared to go. There are all these things you worry about when having your feet washed. Removing your shoes in Western societies can bring out all of these fears that you will reveal sweaty and stinky feet, bunions, callouses, the old nail polish you haven't taken time to remove. Feet have a bad reputation for blemishes.

However, this service deepened my understanding of why taking off your shoes in some cultures communicates that you are standing on sacred ground. At the end of the ritual, the two worship leaders sat down in the chair they used to wash others' feet so that they could meditate for a moment until the music finished. There did not appear to be an opportunity for them to have their own feet washed. Quickly and spontaneously, Wendy, one of the women of New Life who had been living at Diersen for a few months, got up from her seat, walked over to the washing stations, and proceeded to remove the worship leaders' shoes and began to wash their feet. It was a sacred moment, an act of self-giving love.

That moment magnified a reality often hidden by diagnoses and labels as well as the systems and structures of our society. Our very humanity and our survival and flourishing depend on relationships that are far deeper and broader than kinship ties—people and the planet giving to each other. A deeply relational God who continually creates out of chaos calls communities to engage in much more than individual acts of charity, hospitality, and inclusion; God calls for partnership in subduing chaos and creating belonging within communities. Wendy's actions reveal the way we belong together in our blemished bodies as wealthy and poor, leaders and followers, caregivers and needy, doubters and believers, addicted and sober, students and laborers. The last section of the book considers some ways we can work together to advocate for change and to create more communities that pick up and weave the empowerment thread into their daily routines, nurture self-giving love, create belonging, and extend the circle of care for individuals affected by serious mental illness and their families.

CHAPTER SEVEN

Cultivating Belonging and Practicing Intentional Prayer and Advocacy

We have to love and embrace them because their worth is in their creation in the image of God. That is the call to people like me, as a Christian and as a sibling. When there was not rational reason, I had to tap into what is not default human behavior and appeal to that function that is more in the likeness of God. I can love you because you are part of the substance of what makes us all human. That is what the Christian community is called to do.

—Grace

This chapter invites you to think beyond the basic inclusion of people with physical and mental disabilities and their families in congregations and other organizations and to work toward creating nurturing communities of belonging. Stories about people like Wendy, who expressed love and care for others in the ritual of foot washing, remind us that we are all connected. All people, with all their potential and limitations, need to be honored with mutuality and respect. Wendy's expression of caregiving was an act of self-giving love, not demanded or coerced, motivated by guilt or self-interest, or perceived as fulfilling social expectations. In this way, self-giving love is the most basic precondition needed for belonging in community. Authentic relationships require this type of mutuality, reciprocity, and self-giving.

Siblings shared with me in their interviews how the experience of mental illness in their families shaped their concept of community, especially within a church, the body of Christ in the world. Many siblings and

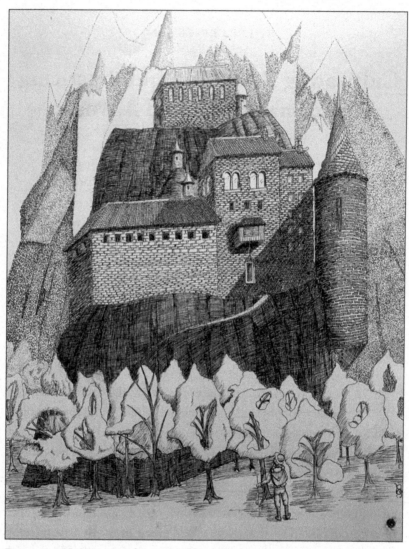

Figure 7.1 *No More Attacks*, a pen-and-ink drawing in a series entitled *Fortress of Solitude* by Chris Hinson. The name of this series comes from the story of Superman. Each drawing expresses the artist's feeling of isolation because of his disability.

other family members with whom I spoke struggled to feel like they fully belonged in a congregation or to a faith tradition. Nearly all expressed conflicted feelings because they encountered some compassionate and charitable responses, but more frequently, they felt isolated. They felt like participants from a distance in the life of the community. They did not have a space to share honestly the chaos they experienced at home or the weight of their family burden and the fears and joys that came along with it. "As for community," Amelia said, "religious institutions are so bad when it comes to mental illness. It is kind of ironic a little bit because all these preachers talk about the trials and tribulations of life but avoid mental illness." Annie had difficulty talking with her pastor about her father's suicide and sister's bipolar disorder: "My pastor said he would be a support person, but he didn't really want to talk. Instead, he encouraged me to work toward self-sufficiency, which made me less transparent and vulnerable about my family's story."

In the last thirty years, a great deal of work has been done by faith and mental health groups to destigmatize mental illness within faith communities, to address the isolation felt by individuals and families, to encourage ministries of presence, and to emphasize the important role that spirituality plays in healing. Noteworthy examples include Pathways to Promise (founded 1988), NAMI FaithNet (founded 1988), Mental Health Ministries (founded 2001), and denominationally based initiatives to educate, train, resource, and support congregations and other faith-based organizations. In addition, a variety of creative and innovative ministries have been developed by local congregations.

The Mental Health and Faith Community Partnership was founded in 2014 by the American Psychiatric Association Foundation and the Interfaith Disability Advocacy Coalition to foster dialogue between psychiatrists and faith leaders. In 2018, this group produced *Mental Health: A Guide for Faith Leaders*, an informative resource that resulted from their dialogues. The guide emphasizes the vital role that religion and spirituality play in helping individuals and caregivers cope, survive, and flourish. Partnership and collaboration among faith leaders, congregations, and mental health professionals are essential to cultivating empowering communities of belonging. Pastors, priests, rabbis, and other leaders within faith communities are often the first people consulted when individuals and families are dealing with mental health and substance abuse issues.

Siblings I interviewed expressed their appreciation for their community of faith by telling stories about times when they felt like their presence in the community mattered and others were willing to walk alongside them and share in caring for and attending to each other's needs. Jade, who was fifteen when I interviewed her, told me that she and her family were living in a small town when her sister was at the height of her struggle with obsessive compulsive disorder and anxiety. At the time, her sister was about seventeen years old. "Our pastor," Jade remembered, "actually had my sister stay at her house and calmed her down. That was one night my mom and I didn't have to worry about her. . . . What I love about the church is that they are a community who will be there, and we will be there for them too." These family members were naming the practices that made them feel a sense of belonging in their church and that the realities they faced on a daily basis were understood. They believed that their presence also increased the good of the community as a whole. Families living with the effects of mental illness require not a specialized ministry but concrete acts of welcome, inclusion, belonging, and love.

My intention in this chapter is to add to the good work that is already being done to advance mental health ministries and companionship and accompaniment movements in congregations and through the many partnerships that exist between faith communities and mental health groups by paying attention to and incorporating the voices of sibling caregivers. In this chapter, I will draw significantly on the work of Erik Carter, the Cornelius Vanderbilt Professor of Special Education at Peabody School of Education of Vanderbilt University, and consider his work in light of the interviews I conducted with siblings and other family members. Carter identifies and explores ten dimensions of belonging that provide the individual threads necessary to begin weaving a social fabric of empowerment for families affected by serious mental illness. I will also offer examples of work being done by congregations and other groups to illustrate strategies that you and the organizations, institutions, and congregations in which you are involved can engage and develop within your own context. It will not be possible to weave a "one size fits all" social fabric to address the circumstances of all individuals affected by serious mental illness and their caregivers. The social fabric of care that is so desperately needed will have to be designed to fit the distinctive circumstances of individuals and caregivers within the communities in which they live.

While I offer some practical strategies and empowering stories here, at the heart of this chapter are really two ecclesiological questions: What do the stories of people with mental illness and the struggles of their families illumine for us about the nature and mission of the church, the body of Christ, in the local community and within a broader society? How can churches clearly articulate the meaning of and embody Jesus's self-giving love in a society that places such a high value on bodies and minds that are considered to be "normal" and prizes the ability to be self-sufficient, efficient, autonomous, and independent? My hope is to move beyond a general description of life-nurturing communities of belonging and call you to act within churches, educational institutions, and other organizations to confront the stigma of serious mental illness, advocate for change, and weave a new social fabric of empowerment.

Committing to More Than Inclusion

Many of the denominational, ecumenical, and interfaith educational resources on disability encourage congregations and other organizations to work toward the full inclusion of individuals affected by physical and mental disabilities and their families. *Inclusion* in this context means being included within a group or structure that already exists. This goal has both positive attributes and significant limitations. Disability and pastoral theologians along with many other educators, psychologists, religious leaders, and social scientists agree that the concept of inclusion is too limiting to foster communities that embrace the full humanity of people with mental and physical impairments.

The concept of inclusion often assumes that people with disabilities can be easily categorized as a homogenous group. However, the term *disability* does not fully encompass the many facets and complexities associated with the human experience of living with chronic health conditions.

Practical theologian John Swinton argues that the "idea of including people with disabilities works on an overly narrow understanding of disability and as such, does not go far enough in overcoming the alienation, stigmatization and exclusion of those whom we choose to name disabled."[1] Swinton calls for a thicker description of the people society labels disabled in order to move beyond thin models of inclusion, which presume that someone is "without a personality or the longings and desires that so-called normal people take for granted."[2]

A second reason that many educators, psychologists, and social scientists urge us to think beyond inclusion is that the practices and policies of existing groups, organizations, and structures are too often defined by norms and values embraced by the dominant society. A commitment to inclusion does not necessarily put the perspectives of people with disabling conditions at the center of group or institutional decision-making and planning. Jason Whitehead, a pastoral theologian at Iliff School of Theology, observes that in churches, cultural values can also "dictate theological beliefs . . . dehumanization in communities of faith and support arise. It is not enough to merely wax poetic about descriptions and meanings; the stigma surrounding persons with mental illness is pervasive, oppressive and permeates communities of faith and support."[3]

In addition, general claims or broad announcements made about inclusion will not necessarily make individuals or families who are minoritized by the dominant society feel welcomed and fully valued. When you live in a society that reduces your identity to a label or diagnosis, lifts up the most able-bodied and able-minded above the rest, and promotes stereotypes of people with severe mental illness, those who are deemed weaker, psycho, or crazy and their families tend to internalize their own inferiority.[4] Remember that studies show that more than half of the news stories presented in the media talk about people with serious mental illness within the context of violent acts. Only about one in seven news stories refers to the successful treatment of serious mental illness.[5] Internalizing the stigma associated with serious mental illness leads to low self-esteem and feelings of shame. Many individuals with serious mental illness may have heard from so many social power brokers that they are unwell, disabled, and will never be able to do meaningful work.

This leads them to feel so disempowered that they cannot advocate for or include themselves in different social groups.

Erik Carter's Ten Dimensions of Belonging

Carter focuses his research and teaching on evidence-based strategies that promote valued roles in school, work, community, and congregational settings for children and adults with intellectual disability, autism, and multiple disabilities. Working with several colleagues, Carter conducted a large-scale, mixed-method research project that interpreted surveys of individuals with intellectual developmental disabilities and their families about ways they can or should flourish within faith communities. I want to clearly recognize that the social experiences and circumstances of individuals affected by intellectual and developmental disabilities and their families may not be exactly the same as those wrestling with serious mental illness. But I also don't want to reinforce the idea that mental illness has more of a stigma—"it is better to be slow than crazy."

Carter introduces his ten dimensions of belonging by suggesting that congregations and other organizations frequently make two initial mistakes when they begin discussions about inclusion. They place too great a focus on the accessibility of physical spaces without considering carefully enough the significant social and attitudinal barriers that people with disabilities face. And they seldom include the perspectives and voices of people with disabilities and their families at the center of their program development. Carter's approach was to listen to people with intellectual and developmental disabilities in order to discover how they name for themselves the dimensions of belonging. The ten dimensions of belonging that were identified included being present and missed, invited, welcomed, known, accepted, supported, cared for, befriended, needed, and loved. Here I will examine these dimensions in light of what I discovered in my own research involving the siblings of people with serious mental illness, many of whom are also caregivers. I also highlight some helpful ways that faith communities and mental health groups are collaborating to weave a stronger social fabric of empowerment.

Being Present and Being Missed

Being present and active and being missed when you are not there are essential dimensions to the experience of belonging within a community of faith, an educational institution, or other organization. Several studies show that the experience of chronic health conditions, disabilities, and functional limitations significantly decreases the likelihood that both adults and children will participate in religious services on a regular basis and increases the prospect that these individuals will never become involved in a community of faith at all. People with chronic health conditions are 9 percent less likely to have ever attended a religious service than their temporarily able-bodied peers.[6] A national study that analyzed participation rates of people with intellectual and developmental disabilities in faith communities found that fewer than half "attended any type of religious service in the prior month."[7]

One of the main reasons for the significant gap in participation in the life of religious communities for people with chronic health conditions, disabilities, and functional limitations is that only 10 percent of congregations report offering some form of support or respite care for families.[8] More than half of parents said that they kept a child from participating due to lack of support. Architecture, attitudes, communication, programs, and the worship experience can all present barriers to full participation for these individuals and their families.

Research focusing specifically on rates of participation of people with serious mental illness and their families in Christian communities is still relatively new and more limited. In 2014, the evangelical research organization Lifeway conducted a national study of evangelical Protestant congregations that incorporated 1,000 telephone and 355 online surveys. Responses to these surveys suggested that another contributing factor to low participation rates was the stigma and shame associated with mental illness.[9]

The Presbyterian Church USA conducted a survey in 2006 of pastors and elders concerning attitudes and the development of congregational programs related to mental illness. Pastors reported that their seminary and other educational training did not equip them to fully include individuals with serious mental illness and their families in congregational life. Ninety-two percent of the respondents did not feel well trained to develop church programs for people with serious mental illness. Seventy-seven percent of respondents did not feel well prepared to provide therapy for these families. Sixty-seven percent did not feel that they had a good understanding of mental illness. Moreover, 61 percent felt ill-equipped even to relate to those with mental illness. Elders who responded to the survey reported that only 16 percent of congregations provide support groups for family members and caregivers of people with serious mental illness. Only 10 percent of congregations held a service of prayer for healing and wholeness. Seven percent of elders had heard a sermon that incorporated themes related to mental illness, and only 4 percent stated that their church advocated for changes in public policies related to mental illness.

It is also important to recognize that experiencing mental health issues as a pastor comes with significant risk. Church employees are excluded from the Americans with Disabilities Act protections provided for workers. Ian Lovett reported in an article published in the *Wall Street Journal* in January 2020 that pastors with mental health problems are frequently fired from their jobs when they disclose these issues. Lovett suggests that this is more common in fundamentalist churches and in congregations where the decision-making authority resides on the local level.[10] In 2012, the Supreme Court ruled in favor of the "ministerial exception" under the guise that it protects religious freedom.

In 2008, the Association of Theological Schools (ATS) studied how institutions welcome people with disabilities and prepare men and women to attend to the unique needs of this constituency. At 91.3 percent of schools, they found that most of the coursework offered related to disability studies and disability theology is in the areas of pastoral care, pastoral theology, and congregational care. About one-fourth of schools never addressed disability studies within historical studies (27.9 percent) or biblical studies (22.4 percent). One-third of the schools did not offer training to prepare religious leaders to work with people with disabilities. At the same time, large percentages of schools indicated that their student bodies included people with learning disabilities (89 percent of schools), physical disabilities

(81.4 percent of schools), emotional and behavioral disabilities (61 percent of schools), and intellectual and developmental disabilities (22.9 percent of schools).[11] Some changes have been made since the ATS issued its challenge in 2008, but programs on disability studies and more specifically disability theology are still too few and far between.[12]

My interviews with siblings of people with serious mental illness revealed another reason for their lack of participation in church: tension may exist when the expectations for participating in the life of a congregation collide with the visible mission of the church, especially if that mission focuses on social issues or countercultural perspectives. Many report that they come to church in order to escape from daily-life issues rather than face pressure to engage more deeply with reality. Family members who provide care for a relative struggling with mental illness are often exhausted and vulnerable. It is not surprising that they often desire a predictable, peaceful, and supportive environment in their faith community.

Mapping Presence and the Story of Sacred Family

Addressing Carter's first dimension (being present and being missed) can begin with a mapping exercise. Congregations and other institutions should map the presence or absence of people with disabilities within their settings. Rebecca Spurrier, assistant professor for worship life and the associate dean for worship at Columbia Seminary, provides a profound and compelling multidimensional and theological portrait of a church in Atlanta, Georgia, that she calls Sacred Family Church. Her book, *The Disabled Church: Human Difference and the Art of Communal Worship*, maps the places, spaces, and rituals through which people in the congregation discover what is sacred in each other.

Sacred Family provides a distinctive context for the type of exploration that Spurrier models because more than half of the members have serious mental illness—schizophrenia, bipolar and anxiety disorders, and cognitive illnesses related to aging. Efforts toward inclusion began at the church in the mid-1990s, when concerns grew among advocates for people with mental illness in the city. Initially, they were concerned for those living on the streets who would need shelter and safe havens during the summer Olympics. The church started a temporary day program called Circle of Friends to address this need. Over time, the program grew beyond its own bounds and into the struggle to become a community "not easily divided into 'us and them'; into people who have mental illness and people who do not; into people who have money and people who do not; into residents of group homes (a greater percentage of whom are Black) and leaders, church visitors and volunteers, and donors (most of whom are white)."[13]

Spurrier maps spaces at Sacred Family where people with serious mental illness are present and where they gather with other members of the congregation. She describes them as relational spaces grounded in self-giving and mutual discovery that transcend the boundaries of social divisions created by charity-oriented models for ministry. Gathering at Sacred Family is not limited to the sanctuary or to a specific day of the week; it does not follow any clearly defined linear progression. People come together in a series of centers that Spurrier calls "sacred refuges"—the parking lot, the garden, picnic tables, the meal hall, the smoking circle, the library, and the sanctuary for noonday prayer, Wednesday Eucharist, and a service called Worship Live. Spurrier observes, "These spaces are sacred refuges not because they are divisively set apart, but because they remain porous to the people who gather within them."[14] Within these spaces, people make room for differences and practice a variety of ways of "sitting, standing, singing, praying, proclaiming, lamenting, and giving thanks together."[15]

Spurrier's description of Sacred Family challenges us to think about where sacred refuges already exist and how to expand them within your own context (see "A Tool for Mapping Spaces, Language, and Rituals within Your School, Organization, or Congregation" at the end of this book).

Being Invited

The stigma surrounding serious mental illness makes it quite possible for those directly affected and their caregivers to navigate the same spaces day after day—or, in the case of congregations, week after week—and never be fully seen, known, accepted, and understood. Whitehead says, "Persons with mental illness are often ghosts that walk among us. From the statistics, what seems clear is that persons living with mental illnesses are all around us, some known, some hidden; the myriad reasons for sharing or hiding their illness, based on what our culture values, should be somewhat obvious."[16] Due to internalized stigma, these individuals and their families may not voluntarily include themselves or respond to broad announcements or invitations.

William Gaventa, the chair of the National Collaborative on Faith and Disability and director of the Summer Institute on Theology and Disability, urges congregations "to begin with a recognition that many people with disabilities and their families will not trust the body of Christ until they have seen and felt it in actions that welcome, affirm, and include."[17] The social amenities churches provide need to invite, give way to, and ensure that deeper conversations are welcomed with these individuals and their families. When I spoke with Annie, she recalled that she went "to church and to weekly Bible study, and there were years it seemed like enough, but I got to a point that it wasn't quite enough. I got to a point that I realized nobody really talked about personal stuff. It was kind of the superficial stuff. How is work? How are your kids doing? I sort of got the idea that I am the only one in this situation. So I learned not to say anything. I was kind of embarrassed and ashamed." In this way, staying on the surface led to silencing Annie, fostering distrust, and reinforcing her feelings of isolation.

A Model of Invitation—Becoming a Caring Congregation

Rev. Susan Gregg-Schroeder, coordinator of Mental Health Ministries, founded the interfaith web-based ministry in 2001 to provide resources to help faith communities destigmatize mental illness. She brings to this task not only pastoral experience but also familiarity with what it is like to live with mental illness.

Gregg-Schroeder had been serving as a pastor of an urban congregation in California for about three years when depression began to overwhelm her. She did not recognize the symptoms at first, but after visiting a psychiatrist, she was admitted to a psychiatric hospital almost immediately. It was the same hospital where she completed her CPE training. Gregg-Schroeder found it difficult to disclose her mental illness to the congregation she served because she feared losing her job. But the senior pastor with whom she worked stood by her. As she put it, "He believed in grace and . . . in me." She first disclosed her struggle in an article for the church newsletter entitled "The Burden of Silence."

Breaking the silence led to educational efforts within the congregation she served, to the creation of a support group for people experiencing depression, and ultimately, to her role in the founding of Mental Health Ministries. Mental Health Ministries introduced the Creating Caring Congregations Model that same year. This five-step plan includes education, commitment or covenant, welcome, support, and advocacy.

Within this model, welcoming involves breaking down barriers that separate people from one another. Some Caring Congregations train members to accompany a person to worship, listen to their stories, or simply help them find quiet spaces within the church building. In addition, inviting people to take leadership roles as liturgists and sharing stories of people and families experiencing serious mental illness in sermons or other programming help destigmatize and normalize their family experiences.

Being Welcomed

Carter stresses that it is not just a matter of "*whether* others know people . . . *how* people with disabilities are known also matters."[18] As discussed earlier, people with disabilities constitute an extremely diverse group and have a rich array of experiences, gifts, and insights they can offer a community. In terms of mental illnesses, experts in disability studies such as Margaret Price urge us to think about *neurodiversity* as opposed to the terms *mental health* and *mental illness* because these terms introduce a dichotomy between wellness and sickness. Identifying people with chronic illness requires some additional negotiating between "the need for solidarity and diversity."[19] The language we use is an important element of true welcome.

People-First Language and Sidewalk Ministries—Ways to Welcome

Individuals and caregivers must have opportunities and spaces to name, claim, and share their own stories. Adopting people-first language as an intentional practice is an important way to welcome. Other terms people use to name their experiences include *mental health service user/consumer, psychiatric system survivor, neurotypical,* and *neurodiversity*. At Sacred Family Church, "people are not known by their particular diagnoses and . . . seldom represent their lives as unusual."[20] A number of schools, institutions, and organizations are also opting to use phrases like *accessibility services* rather than *disability services* to emphasize human potentialities and promise rather than limitations.

Another way to nurture human connection and to welcome individuals affected by serious mental illness and their families is to set up a "listening post." Pastor Barbara F. Meyers and Karolyn Stenlund, both spiritual directors, began a Sidewalk Listening Post in the East Bay area of San Francisco for the purpose of listening to the most vulnerable in their community and as part of their mental health ministry. Meyers and Stenlund began their collaborative ministry by integrating the concept of a listening post introduced by Marcia Wakeland after completing the training offered by Sidewalk-Talk.[21] Their ministry involves setting up folding chairs on the sidewalk and welcoming others to sit with them and share their stories—including their hopes and haunts, dreams and disappointments. The primary goal of Sidewalk-Talk is as simple as it is profound—to challenge a culture driven by efficiency and busyness by nurturing human connection through meaningful listening in public areas.

Being Known

Mental illness is treated, understood, and judged so differently by society than physical illness that the burden of explaining the nature of mental illness is often placed on the individuals and family members. Amelia, a young woman whom I interviewed, dealt with a medical condition that led to a severe bout of depression. She commented, "Physical conditions and physical impairments are definitely visible. People have to see it to believe it. . . . You know how you can hold a toy in front of a baby and then put it behind your back and they think it ceases to exist? That is exactly how I think people deal with mental illness." A parent who took part in a national survey focusing on barriers to participation in congregational life further observed, "We wish we had a community to belong to, however . . . we have not had the time or energy to seek out and prepare (educate) a new spiritual home for ourselves."[22]

Siblings and other relatives with whom I spoke repeatedly mentioned that having a family member with serious mental illness "changes everything about how the family functions." Jade said, "You can't really understand unless you have lived it, and it was just kind of hard because it felt like no one really understood what was going on in our family's life." Hurdles often need to be overcome just to complete ordinary tasks. A parent reflected, "Do I work? Do I not work?" and talked about wondering whether others "have been through what we have been through." He was always questioning, "Is it safe to share our story? Is it safe to take our daughter to youth group or not?"

Behavioral attributes associated with some intellectual and developmental disabilities and mental illnesses such as a lack of social inhibitions and impulse control can also come into conflict with church culture. A hidden agenda of social conduct exists in most congregations. Children with anxiety, autism, developmental delays, depression, speech problems, and brain injury all report lower odds of ever attending religious services in comparison to their temporarily able-bodied peers. Most siblings whom I interviewed recognized that it can be difficult for church communities to welcome and embrace their family members with serious mental illness. Glenn admitted that his "brother has struggled in churches in being welcomed and received. I struggle with this too because I believe church should be a place where someone with mental illness can be embraced and cared for, but I also know how draining my brother can be, and he is awkward and difficult to be with."

Emotional Support, Service Animals, and Animal Therapy at Church

Churches, synagogues, mosques, and other places of worship are exempt from the American with Disabilities Act laws (though maybe not from state laws) that require them to allow emotional support or service animals. But interfaith and mental health groups, as well as denominational mental health ministries and networks such as the United Church of Christ, Unitarian Universalist Church, and the Anabaptist Disabilities Network, encourage faith communities not to claim this exemption.

Reese, one of the young women I interviewed, deals with anxiety. She emphasized that animals provide a good coping mechanism facing different environments, particularly when she experiences anxiety. She and her family suggest that allowing or providing emotional support animals at church "gives her more peace of mind" and helps her feel welcomed, received, and known.

Increasingly, colleges and universities are allowing emotional support and service animals on campus as a result of student petitions. Many universities and colleges also bring therapy dogs to campus to help with the anxiety and stress that students experience during exams.

St. James United Church of Christ in Havertown, Pennsylvania, offers an example of how a congregation began a pet therapy ministry. In 2018, they developed a partnership with PAWS for People, a pet therapy organization in the mid-Atlantic region. They wanted to focus their ministry on four key areas: helping individuals and families dealing with addiction, alleviating the stress experienced by people undergoing cancer treatment, supporting the LGBTQIA community, and developing a pet therapy program to help children and developmentally disabled adults. The congregation is a PAWS training facility and now has three dogs and several human volunteers. Volunteers in the congregation bring their therapy dogs to hour-long reading sessions for elementary students. Churches and other faith communities might also consider such a practice during the holiday season, when many people experience a heightened sense of loneliness.[23]

An Additional Spiritual Dimension to Being Known

The siblings and other family members whom I interviewed are all actively involved in a faith community. Their participation provides a distinctive opportunity to understand how serious mental illness affects religious belief and one's experience in a congregational setting. They expressed a need for deeper theological conversations and an additional spiritual dimension to being known. In our conversations, several theological themes consistently emerged: the meaning and purpose of serious mental illness, the struggle to deal with mental health issues in the context of fundamentalist Christianity, the fear of not being seen as a "good" family, the guilt placed on families because of traditional Christian teachings on suicide, and the shame felt by caregivers who question how much they can personally sacrifice when they take on that role in our society.

Sarah Griffith Lund, a sibling and minister in the United Church of Christ in Florida, makes some powerful observations about how her family's experience of mental illness shapes her brother's and her own theology. Her brother, Scott, "testifies that his faith is shaped by his mental health . . . when he is stable he believes in God; when he is feeling manic he believes he is God; and when he is feeling depressed he believes there is no God." She continues, "My brother did not make the cross of mental illness, but it is still his to bear. As his sister, it is mine to bear too. By bearing the cross of mental illness and carrying it, we can move it—not rid ourselves of it or deny—to a place of transformation like Golgotha. On that hill the cross became something not to be despised but a thing to transform the world."[24]

Being understood personally and spiritually requires embracing serious mental illness and mental health as more than topics for discussion or regarding people with disabilities as objects of compassion, charity, and sympathy. Faith communities can lend a powerful witness by providing spaces for sharing stories. They can make room for those living with chronic health conditions and proclaim the ways that people with mental and physical impairments embody Jesus's alternative social logic.

Empowering Liturgy, Ritual, and Preaching

Kathy Black, a professor of homiletics at Claremont School of Theology, asserts that one of the first steps for able-bodied people who preach and sit in the pews is to work together on overcoming their own fear of disabling conditions. Black says, "It is a very frightening thing to feel out of control of one's own thoughts, behavior, and even identity."[25] She suggests that our "fear is often the greatest barrier to healing—both for those who need the healing and for those who offer a helping hand."[26]

Black calls on religious leaders to bridge the gap between ancient views of healing and modern medicine, to avoid "hermeneutical hazards" associated with interpretations of narratives that associate healing with cure, and to promote a "theology of interdependence." Black explores the approach of examining and altering the implicit and explicit use of images and descriptions of conditions that connect disability with sin in liturgies, rituals, Bible studies, and sermons. This practice can be transformative as it invites congregations to think about the social construction of disability in church and society and how individuals and families internalize these stereotypes. It is important to show richer character development of people with disabling conditions named in the biblical text and to emphasize how God works "to transform our lives at every moment, in all our various circumstances, through the power of love."[27]

Rituals, liturgies, and sermons are a tremendous source of comfort when they emphasize that mental illness "is not caused by lack of faith or spiritual commitment." A wide variety of online resources have been produced by denominational, ecumenical, and interfaith groups to support networking and provide models for services of healing and wholeness, including Mental Health Prayer Days or Mental Health Sundays, Caregiver Sundays, as well as examples of sermons on mental health issues.

Being Accepted

Creating room for individuals affected by serious mental illness and their families within congregational and other settings will also mean that things won't and can't always proceed in a programmatic way. Grace, one of the siblings introduced earlier, wanted to share what her family's struggle to cope with her brother's schizophrenia had taught her about her own spirituality. She began, "For many years, we thought what we identified as strange and disruptive behaviors related to his addiction to alcohol and marijuana." Grace described her brother, Will, as the "clown of the town." At one point, Will had a mental breakdown and ended up in a psychiatric unit. The family traveled to the hospital to be with him and felt traumatized by the experience. When he was released from the hospital, care for Will fell on their parents' shoulders. Grace and Will's father is a pastor. The congregation felt compassion for the family, supported Will and Grace's parents, and dealt with Will's bizarre behaviors by normalizing them. Grace said they were compassionate, but they lacked the training and capacity to deal with the reality of Will's mental illness.

When their father died, Grace insisted on an open casket for the funeral at the church. When the family filed into the sanctuary at the beginning of the service, Will began crying uncontrollably. He climbed into the casket to lie down with his father a few moments later. No one really knew exactly how to respond. Eventually, Grace consoled her brother and was able to persuade him to leave the sanctuary for a moment to collect himself. She had intended to offer comments in honor of her father's life, but when she was able to return to the sanctuary, the time for sharing memories had ended, and she missed the opportunity. For Grace, the congregation's expectations for what a "normal" funeral ritual is and should be took precedence over her need to share words of remembrance on behalf of her father. When thinking about her brother's experience, Grace observed, "The reality is that to belong together with crazy people, you need to open yourself up to the ways that other people surprise you and make room for things that are imperfect and constantly chaotic, even in your theology and the church."

Designating Spaces to Calm the Storm

People with serious mental illness and their siblings and other relatives who also serve as caregivers may have distinct needs and different gifts regarding engaging in communal activities, religious practices, or other rituals. One parent with whom I spoke observed, "We need to raise questions particularly in congregational settings about how music and lights and loud noises create anxiety for some people. They can impact kids with mental illness. You can watch kids start to melt down just in the course of worship. The big question for me as a parent is, How do we balance what the majority needs out of the service with what kids struggling with anxiety issues might need? Most who struggle with anxiety and other mental illnesses are longing for relationships and connections more than the teaching, singing, and the lessons."

There is so much going on in the daily lives of families affected by serious mental illness that cultivating silence and intentional practices of daily meditation and contemplative prayer are life-sustaining. All but one of the siblings whom I interviewed mentioned the need for silence. Glenn said, "Practices that sustain me are just being quiet, journaling, [and] the prayer of examen once a week. They offer a way to process everything that is going on in my life."

Being Supported

Carter emphasizes that the "ordinary supports congregations provide to any member should also be extended to families impacted by disability"[28]—namely, childcare, transportation, small groups, and financial assistance. However, the circumstances of individuals affected by serious mental illness and their families are distinct. For this reason, they require additional support to enable their full participation in the life of a congregation or other organizations. This may include such things as building or supporting mutual aid societies, intentionally designing mentoring programs, and providing housing assistance.

Mutual Aid Societies and Mentoring—Assistance Congregations Can Provide outside the Mainstream

Mutual aid societies are grassroots organizations that form to support the needs of communities that do not have access to traditional lending institutions. The Free African Society in Philadelphia was first in the United States and formed in 1787 under the leadership of Richard Allen and Absalom Jones, both clergy and abolitionists. Allen later founded the African Methodist Episcopal Church, and Jones led an interracial congregation at St. George's Methodist Episcopal Church in Philadelphia. The society's mission was to support Black people within a nation ruled by white supremacy. Mutual aid societies and informal lending circles became a significant source of support for immigrants throughout the nineteenth and early twentieth centuries.

These groups can be organized to provide financial aid and benefits. For people living in vulnerable positions, mutual aid societies can become networks for support in terms of services and other activities. One important principle is that everyone has a voice in the decision-making process and the opportunity to receive benefits. Recently, mutual aid societies are being used as a way for people with disabilities faced with health care rationing during the COVID-19 crisis to band together to provide assistance for one another. For example, the Disability Justice Culture Club prioritized the needs of elderly Black, brown, and other people of color in Oakland, California, due to the "eugenic approaches to healthcare" that emerged during the pandemic.[29]

Mentoring is greatly needed on a variety of levels. The lack of appropriate and effective support and rehabilitation for employment contributes significantly to high rates of unemployment for people with serious mental illness. However, employment provides much more than supplemental income; it is also a means of social inclusion, building self-confidence, and extending one's network of support. Congregations and other faith-based groups have long served as job networking organizations. Expanding this form of mentoring to address the specific needs of people with serious mental illness would provide much-needed help for many families.

Several sibling caregivers referenced the challenges they faced in navigating the mental health system and their invisibility within the system. Faith communities could draw on their own human resources (social workers, lawyers, mental health professionals, teachers, etc.) to create and publicly post a list of community organizations that assist individuals and families affected by serious mental illness. Faith communities could sponsor a disability justice fair during Mental Health Awareness month (May) where these human resources come together to share information and give advice to individuals and their caregivers.

Being Cared For

Family members provide 80 percent of long-term care needs in the United States, and most of their labor in this area is unpaid, putting caregivers themselves at risk. Respite care provides a greatly needed break for people who serve others in this way and can improve their overall mental and physical health. Government-funded agencies offer limited types of respite care for individuals affected by chronic health conditions and serious mental illness and their families. Waiting lists are often very lengthy. Studies show that only about 8 percent of families have access to respite care. Seventy-five percent of families with children with special needs from birth to the age of seventeen have unmet needs for respite care. This is a staggering care gap for these individuals and families. At the same time, fewer than 10 percent of congregations offer any kind of respite care for families affected by physical and mental disabilities. Addressing this care gap would create meaningful ties to the surrounding community and foster a sense of belonging within a congregational setting.

Dana Dillon is a Roman Catholic moral theologian and a supportive caregiver for her brother, Paul, who has serious mental illness. She draws on the concept of the common good from Catholic social thought to provide a theological basis for the mutual support that families and churches should provide for an individual with serious mental illness. Dillon says,

> Presenting the common good as the good of each person and the good of all persons, [Catholic social teaching] relies upon the intrinsically communal nature of the person, as evidenced in the shared goods of the family. In fact, the work of the family to support a member with a mental health condition is an excellent image of the way that the good of one person and the good of all people is interconnected. Even as the family turns within to support the flourishing of its ill, vulnerable member, it turns outward to advocate for the resources required for this work.[30]

The larger faith community plays a vital role in supporting the family and the person with mental illness, which in turn enables the church "to support all persons and families with these (and other, similar) vulnerabilities better."[31]

Some Ways Congregations Close the Care Gap

More traditional approaches to closing the care gap could include visiting with and taking food to individuals and caregivers dealing with a mental health crisis and providing day programming for adults and children with physical and mental impairments. Some congregations also develop respite care programs that aim to avoid perpetuating the stigma associated with intellectual and developmental disabilities and serious mental illness through children's buddy programs that are inclusive of all children. Another less common approach is creating a time bank. A time bank provides for a system of bartering that allows people to invest their time in exchange for goods or services that others can provide. It is driven by values that emphasize that everyone has assets to share, caregiving is also a form of work, reciprocity

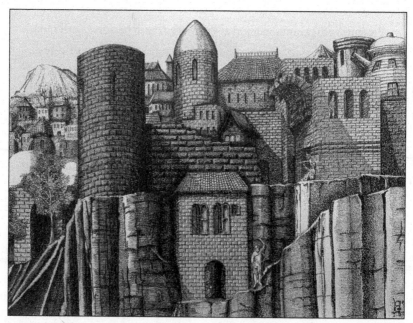

Figure 7.2 *Traders Outpost*, another pen-and-ink drawing in a series entitled *Fortress of Solitude* by Chris Hinson.

is empowering, and building a social network is important to the community as a whole.

Being Befriended

Carter emphasizes that friendship that embodies values of "companionship, intimacy, reciprocity, and support . . . can be vital to one's thriving."[32] Spiritual friendship has been central to Christian identity from the very beginning, but we are losing this art in US society. In the United States, trends toward individualization and social isolation are compounded by prosperity theology, which celebrates material wealth and ideal physical and mental health as evidence of God's blessing. Thus many communities of faith are abdicating their responsibility to accompany others in their physical and emotional challenges. Ethicist Ramón Luzárraga rightly points out that too many US Christians hope to resolve suffering from physical or mental illness by calling for a simple show of faith, while Jesus's story teaches us that God enters into solidarity with us, embraces our human vulnerabilities and limitations, and accompanies us along the way.[33]

All this being said, many communities of faith see their ministry as one of mutual consolation and support for those who are burdened by illness and difficulties of all kinds. Programs have been developed to train community members to listen to and befriend those who are isolated or struggling.

Companionship—Pathways to Promise

Accompaniment and companionship movements arise among communities of people living in circumstances where they are suspended somewhere between destitution and survival. The journey begins with the acknowledgment that all human beings have inherent value and worth and share the common experience of depending on each other and the planet for their own survival.

Rev. Craig Rennebohm began to develop the model of companionship in 1987 after witnessing how the care gap

impacted people with serious mental illness who were released
from the hospital after receiving acute care. Many ended up on
the streets of Seattle, Washington, Rennebohm's hometown.
Companionship is about a ministry of presence and developing
relationships that are supportive and grounded in mutuality,
reciprocity, and kindness. The spiritual practices of companionship
include hospitality, neighboring, journeying side-by-side, listening,
and accompaniment.

Rennebohm and David Paul share stories about the
beginnings of the companionship movement in their book *Souls
in the Hands of a Tender God: Stories of the Search for Home and
Healing on the Streets*. Mental Health Chaplaincy offered the first
companionship training to members of Plymouth United Church
of Christ in Seattle more than thirty years ago. The congregation
first formed a companionship team to welcome people who came
to worship in distress. Later, they worked with Rennebohm to
found the Plymouth House of Healing, an emergency housing
and respite program for people recently discharged from inpatient psychiatric treatment after a mental health crisis. Their
approach is informed by Rennebohm's study of family care in
European cities such as Geel, Belgium, and Bobigny, a suburb of
Paris, France. Rennebohm says that "family care 'normalizes' the
illness experience"[34] because people are welcomed without being
judged.

Communities of faith continue to be trained in the model of
companionship through a partnership between Mental Health
Chaplaincy and Pathways to Promise.

Being Needed

Authentic relationships involve reciprocity and the recognition that
everyone is needed and has gifts to bring. Carter says that many churches
are now "recognizing the importance of 'ministry to' people with disabilities, [but] many still struggle to move toward the place of 'ministry
by' people with disabilities. People with intellectual and developmental

disabilities are still viewed as the 'designated recipients' of service and outreach; the roles of giver and receiver remain strikingly static."[35] Asking what gifts individuals with serious mental illness and their caregivers bring to congregational and communal life is essential to belonging.

There are important theological reasons why faith communities need to shift their perception in this way. Recognizing the gifts that people with mental and physical disabilities bring to a congregation carries along with it a new way of seeing the divine within others. People with disability are also living out their faith and are vessels for wisdom. One of the primary goals of religious institutions—congregations, schools, colleges, seminaries, and so on—is to invite people into community to live out their Christian vocations. The idea of vocation may relate to one's form of employment, but more deeply, vocation reflects the gifts and talents that each individual is given by God. Finding ways for everyone to utilize those gifts celebrates and honors God's continual creative activity in our world.

Master Artists and Mentors

Bridgehaven is a mental health program in Louisville, Kentucky, founded in 1963 by the local chapter of the National Council of Jewish Women, before the formation of community mental health centers. It is the third non-hospital-based program in the United States to treat disorders such as schizophrenia and bipolar using a community-based model. Art therapy plays an important role in Bridgehaven's program. Opportunities are offered during the year for members of the local community to attend art shows and purchase the work done by people in the recovery program at Bridgehaven. Supporting artists learning to cope with mental health issues contributes to individual and communal health.

Individuals who are affected by serious mental illness and their caregivers can also be key mentors for others. The concept of peer mentoring can be traced back to the era of *traitment moral* in France and has been advanced more recently through recovery movements and grassroots self-help initiatives that began in the

1970s in the United States. Many mental health organizations and ministries offer mentor training opportunities for people with serious mental illness who have learned to cope with and navigate the system.

Family members, especially siblings who serve as caregivers, also need mentors and friends who have lived through similar situations. Members help them understand how to navigate complex relationships and family dynamics and find the social services, supports, and programs that are available in the local community. As parents age or die, siblings face distinct challenges as caregivers. For example, those in the sandwich generation find themselves trying to care for their own children as well as aging parents. Throw in the burden of also caring for a sibling with serious mental illness, and the sandwich effect intensifies. Those who are willing and able to take on caregiving responsibilities remain largely invisible to counseling professionals, the medical community, and government agencies. Finding mentors from families who have dealt with similar situations along the way is essential to the caregiver's own survival, well-being, and navigation through the mental health system.

The National Alliance on Mental Illness (NAMI) is well known for providing some excellent programming on family-to-family and peer-to-peer opportunities that can be offered within local churches. Support for these services could be given simply by offering to provide space. In addition, congregations and other organizations could develop a sib-to-sib network where siblings would have a safe place to tell their own stories, normalize their family experiences, and share what they have learned about navigating the mental health system.

Being Loved

Individuals with developmental and intellectual disabilities clearly identify being loved as the tenth dimension of belonging, but Carter observes that "social scientists working in this area have been largely silent on love."[36] The theological tradition, however, has much to say about the many forms of love. When Jesus reflects on the greatest commandment in the teachings of the Torah in the Gospel of Matthew, he says, "*You must love the Lord your God with all your heart, with all your being,* and with all your mind. This is the first and greatest commandment. And the second is like it: *You must love your neighbor as you love yourself.* All the Law and the Prophets depend on these two commands" (Matthew 22:37–40). Loving your neighbor as yourself begins by seeing and embracing the fullness of their humanity.

Francisco Argüelles Paz y Puente, the executive director of the Living Hope Wheelchair Association in Houston, Texas, has been part of grassroots movements in solidarity with people with disabilities for decades. Living Hope Wheel Chair Association emphasizes accompaniment and advocacy. It was formed in 2005 after the Harris County Hospital District in Houston stopped providing medical supplies to the uninsured. Many of the people who lacked insurance were migrant workers who needed medical supplies because they became disabled after enduring spinal cord injuries while laboring in the fields or while working on construction sites around the area. Paz y Puente says, "Here we were in Houston, a city that is home to the largest medical centre in the world, and a group of men and women who broke their backs helping build this city were faced with a crisis of survival."[37] In response to the forced scarcity of resources, people "chose to organize themselves, selling flowers in the streets, raffling TVs in churches, organizing car washes, and selling food to gather resources and buy medical supplies that they would then share among themselves. . . . Now, fourteen years later, Living Hope is able to distribute enough catheters, diapers, and wheelchairs to anyone who shows up to our monthly supplies distribution day, including a growing number of US citizens."[38]

For Paz y Puente, "accompaniment is never about parachuting in to save 'the other.' It is not about discovering an issue, problem, or community, and then colonizing it, jumping to propose solutions that reduce the people to a problem without asking for their own definition of the problem or their ideas for solutions."[39] He says that ultimately, what accompaniment is all about is *mutual rehumanization*—learning to see beyond stigma and the attitudes that divide, discovering together an authentic and deep love for each other, and working collaboratively to establish the conditions for individuals with disabilities and their families to cope, survive, and thrive.

Advocacy

Advocacy is a central part of expressing love for individuals affected by serious mental illness and their families. Many of the justice issues named in this book involve basic human rights and gaps in public policy. There are a variety of ways that churches can partner with established advocacy groups.

The Creating Caring Congregations Model suggests attending workshops and conferences on mental health issues and contacting your elected representatives or visiting them as a group. In addition, they encourage supporting candidates running for public office who are working on mental health issues. Further, they recommend keeping in contact with advocacy and training groups such as NAMI, Depression and Bipolar Support Alliance (DBSA), Mental Health Ministries, Pathways to Promise, and Mental Health America (MHA). Participating in community events such as mental health walks highlights the issue within your local community.

My interviews with siblings and my conversations with leaders working in this area in my community also revealed other places where advocacy is needed to address gaps in policy. Clinical psychologist and mental health advocate Sheila Schuster said that ongoing efforts are needed to ensure that mental health care receives the same benefits as physical health care. She argued that the number of beds in crisis stabilization units should be proportional to the population of a particular region. She also mentioned educating the community about the distinctive needs of people with co-occurring conditions and increasing financial support through programs such as Social Security Disability Income (SSDI).

Other advocacy work directly relates to caregivers. For example, when someone is unable to stay on medication and experiences a crisis, sometimes the only way caregivers can get that family member the treatment they need is through a mental inquest warrant, which leads to involuntary commitment. A wider variety of avenues and greater visibility for caregivers (including siblings) within the mental health system that do not involve court intervention are needed. In addition, some states offer special services to support people with intellectual disabilities and their caregivers. These programs offer significant financial aid to allow people with intellectual disabilities to live in their local community. The support can be used for personal care, behavioral support, camps, and respite care for caregivers. In Kentucky and several other states, additional financial assistance can be applied for through the Michelle P. Waiver (MPW) program. Comparable services should be developed for individuals affected by serious mental illness and their families.

Gathering Threads of Empowerment

At some point in our lives, nearly all of us will experience a physically, mentally, or emotionally disabling condition. Disability impacts more than twenty-one million families in the United States; that means that one in four families has at least one relative with a disability of some sort at the present time. Disability is a normal part of the human experience, and yet our social institutions continue to treat the experience as if it is an exception to the rule.

People with serious mental illness and their families are some of the most vulnerable people in society, and their lived experiences raise critically important and perennial questions for people of faith as we continue to envision how to embody Christ's countercultural social logic. Numerous studies show that the vast majority of people with disabilities in the United States remain unchurched and absent from congregations. Jesus challenged social hierarchies defined by elite views of ideal forms and norms for human minds and bodies. His ministry modeled accompanying those who had been exiled from community and set adrift. He embraced living in self-giving love, entering into and calming the storms of chaos, and empowering the most vulnerable to confront attitudes, beliefs, systems, and structures that valued people according to their social utility rather than celebrating their creation in God's image. The church, as the body of Christ in the world, bears tremendous potential for good. As a social institution, it can advocate for an alternative vision of authentic community that embodies Jesus's self-giving love. Paul wrote, "If all were one and the same body part, what would happen to the body? But as it is, there are many parts but one body. So the eye can't say to the hand, 'I don't need you,' or in turn, the head can't say to the feet, 'I don't need you.' Instead, the parts of the body that people think are the weakest are the most necessary" (1 Corinthians 12:19–22).

The knitting community at my church still gives me tremendous hope because it continues to create fabric that can be stretched or tightened according to the needs of the body who will be using it—tiny newborn bodies, sick bodies, healthy bodies, bodies with broken bones, healing bodies, dying bodies, bodies transitioning in relationships or moving to new spaces and places, bodies with minds that have thoughts like tornadoes, and bodies that are exhausted by caregiving. Handcrafted knitted fabric pieces symbolize that we are all bound together and belong to each other as one in the body of Christ. The stories told in these pages by and about people struggling with mental illness and their family caregivers must do more than bring these experiences out of the crawl spaces of individual households and churches. Their voices call us to witness to the injustices faced by people with serious mental illness and their families, to cry out for a "mutual rehumanization" in our society, and to act prophetically to reorient the nature and mission of churches to partner with many other institutions in weaving a social fabric of empowerment.

Additional Resources

Questions for Individual Reflection or Group Discussion

Introduction

1. What is dutiful love and how does it connect to Christian concepts of self-sacrificial love in the introduction? Discuss or take note of feminist, womanist, and other critiques of the concept of self-sacrifice. Do you agree with these scholars that self-sacrifice is a troubling concept even in the abstract? Why or why not?
2. Has your religious community emphasized self-sacrifice as an ideal? If so, in what ways?
3. Reflect in writing or in your discussion group on your own experiences of caregiving. Do you expect that your responsibilities to care for others will extend over the course of a lifetime? If so, what are the challenges you are confronting or think you will confront? When is caregiving a joy and fulfillment of duty? When have you felt like caregiving leaves you feeling depleted?

Part I: Heading into Households and Crawl Spaces

Chapter One: Being Parents and Children in a Culture of Stigma and Shame

1. Labeling is one of the issues raised in this chapter. Terms used to name and describe disabilities are not neutral. Think about or discuss how the concept of disability can be used to discriminate against certain groups. How does the stigma associated with disability shape interactions that individuals and families have with

key power groups such as teachers, landlords, mental health and other medical professionals, and religious leaders?

2. What did you learn from the stories told by individuals and parents about internalized stigma?

3. How does religion inform concepts of the good family and contribute to and perpetuate the stigma associated with serious mental illness?

Chapter Two: Siblings Naming Their Own Experiences

1. Were there surprises for you in the stories told by siblings in this chapter? What distinctive challenges do people face when they become caregivers for a sibling with serious mental illness?

2. Reflect on the ways that siblings describe how their relationship with a brother or sister expanded their own sense of mutuality, agency, love, and community. How did they describe God's activity in the midst of their experiences?

3. If serious mental illness affects your family, where do you see that the social fabric of care has unraveled in the United States and in your local community?

4. What has been your experience in your community of faith of attention and support given to families affected by serious mental illness?

Part II: History and Current Circumstances

Chapter Three: A Brief Overview of the Treatment of People with Serious Mental Illness in the US Context

1. Jews, Muslims, heretics, witches, and people with mental and physical conditions that were considered disabling threatened the social hierarchy of the Middle Ages. Observations regarding Western European policies intended to maintain the "health" and well-being of the body politic and the church made by historians such as Nicholas Terpstra will be important in deepening our understanding of the

treatment of people with mental and physical impairments through the twentieth century. Reflect on your understanding of why these groups came to be understood as pollutants or threats to the health of the body politic and the body of Christ and how those ideas influenced European colonizers of North America.

2. Discuss the historical importance of the creation of state-supported psychiatric hospitals or asylums. What were they intended to provide for people with serious mental illness? Ultimately, why do you think they failed?

3. How did Christian communities play a role in supporting the eugenics movements in the United States and Europe? What responsibility do you think religious leaders have today to explore the connections between Christian concepts and eugenics movements and to apologize for involvement in them?

4. Reflect on Anton Boisen's experience as a survivor of treatment in a psychiatric hospital and how that informed his approach to theological education and the training of pastoral leaders. Why was it essential to Boisen to connect theological reflection to "living human documents"?

Chapter Four: Prescription for Poverty

1. Why are there higher rates of poverty, homelessness, and potential jail time among people with serious mental illness? Identify at least three systemic and structural causes of poverty named and discussed within this chapter.

2. Where do you see the greatest care gap in your local community?

3. Some scholars suggest that increasing the likelihood of employment among people with serious mental illness requires training programs and creating more flexible work environments. Can you imagine or have you encountered a work environment that would allow for people struggling with mental health issues to increase their income, develop much-needed social networks, and contribute to a larger community? If so, describe the characteristics of that work environment.

4. The chapter ends with Eleanor and Christina's story. How do these two sisters help you understand the vulnerability of people with serious mental illness? Do other stories come to mind that you are interested in reflecting on or sharing with others?

Part III: Empowerment, Alternatives, and Advocacy

Chapter Five: Biblical Threads of Empowerment

1. Consider the social construction of disability in the Greco-Roman world. How were bodily differences and one's state of mental health used to affirm the power and privilege of the social elite?

2. What is physiognomy? How do Jesus and Paul confront physiognomy and the ordering of the household in the ancient world?

3. Reflect on the empowerment thread traced in this chapter. How are people with mental and physical impairments in the biblical stories included here seen as empowering agents of change?

4. Adair, one of the siblings whom I interviewed, talked about needing a "God who can do triage every day." How can reading and interpreting the biblical narrative with the experiences of individuals affected by serious mental illness and their siblings in mind be empowering to these families?

Chapter Six: Communities of Empowerment and Belonging

1. Have you witnessed or personally accompanied someone in the midst of a struggle with serious mental illness? What did you learn from the experience?

2. Identify the shared norms, values, and practices of the individuals and communities discussed in this chapter. What do the convent at Rupertsberg, Bethel, Geel, L'Arche, and Diersen House have in common?

Chapter Seven: Cultivating Belonging and
Practicing Intentional Prayer and Advocacy

1. Consider the limitations of inclusion discussed in this chapter. How do you define the distinction between inclusion and belonging? In what ways does your church, school, or other organizations in which you are involved nurture belonging?

2. Four reasons for low participation rates in religious services and Christian congregations are identified in this chapter. Reflect on the presence or absence of people with mental and physical disabilities in the church, school, or other organizations in which you are involved. What limits or may enhance participation rates?

3. Fewer than 10 percent of congregations offer respite care programs to support individuals and caregivers dealing with chronic health conditions. What creative approaches to respite care programs can you imagine your congregation working collaboratively to develop?

4. This chapter identifies the importance of mentoring. What types of mentoring have been most beneficial to you, a family member, or friend struggling with mental health issues? What are some ways to cultivate good mentoring relationships and develop programs in your church, educational institution, or other organizations?

Questions Asked during Interviews of Siblings and Other Family Members Affected by Serious Mental Illness

1. Please share your age or your age range. The reason for this is to identify the era of care for people with mental illness that would have shaped your family's response. I will not share your age in the book.
2. How would you like to be named in the book? Please choose a pseudonym that can be used in public reporting on this project.
3. How do you name or describe your gender and your own racial ethnic identity?
4. Explain the details of your experience of mental illness within your family and any information regarding that experience you think is relevant to the study.
5. Did you or do you experience "secondary stigmatization" as a sibling and family member of someone with mental illness? If so, in what ways?
6. How did you first learn about mental illness in your family? Was it talked about openly or not?
7. How have you and your relatives planned for the care of people with mental illness in your family? What obstacles have you or your family faced in arranging for care?
8. Has your experience of mental illness impacted or shaped your faith and belief? If so, in what ways?
9. How has your experience of mental illness shaped your concept of community, especially within your church, synagogue, or mosque?
10. What theological concepts, specific religious practices, and/or rituals sustain you and are liberating through your experience of traveling with family members who have a mental illness?

11. Are there theological concepts, specific religious practices, and/or rituals that are problematic in light of your experience of mental illness in your family?

12. Do you think any circumstances would be different if your family member(s) had suffered from a physical disease as opposed to a disease of the mind? Why or why not?

13. Do you have any other comments or observations you would like to add?

Timeline of Significant Events Related to Policy Shifts, Treatment, and Attitudes toward Mental Illness from the Mid-twentieth Century to the Present

1935 FDR signs the Social Security Act into law. The act does not include a national health insurance plan.

1942 Congress passes the Stabilization Act, which limits employer wage increases in order to fight wartime inflation. Businesses first begin offering employer-sponsored health insurance.

1943 The Wagner-Murray-Dingell Bill proposes universal health care for all through payroll taxes. Additional proposals are made throughout the 1940s but are challenged as socialist. During this same year, a group of conscientious objectors working in state mental hospitals reports the inhumane conditions in state asylums.

1945 Congressional hearings open to consider the National Neuropsychiatric Institute and the National Mental Health Plan.

1946 *Life Magazine* publishes "Bedlam 1946," an exposé covering the mistreatment of mentally ill patients in Pennsylvania's Byberry Hospital and Ohio's Cleveland State. In July, Congress passes the National Mental Health Act.

1949 The National Institute of Mental Health (NIMH) is created. Portuguese neurologist Egas Moniz wins the Nobel Prize in Physiology or Medicine for developing the lobotomy procedure.

1952 Dwight Eisenhower's presidential campaign platform includes opposition to national health insurance. Under Eisenhower, national health insurance receives little attention. The American Psychiatric Association (APA) publishes the *Diagnostic and Statistical Manual of Mental Disorders* (DSM), the first official manual to classify mental disorders for clinical use.

1954   The APA cosponsors with then senator John F. Kennedy a call for a national commission to assess the state of mental health care in the United States and to develop a national plan. During the same year, the Food and Drug Administration (FDA) approves Thorazine to treat psychotic episodes, an alternative to electroshock therapy and the lobotomy procedure. About fifteen antipsychotic drugs are introduced in the United States between 1954 and 1975.

1955   The number of patients in public mental health hospitals reaches a record high of 558,000. The deinstitutionalization movement begins this same year as Congress passes the Mental Health Study Act to establish a commission to evaluate the nation's mental health system.

1960   The US government begins tracking national health expenditures for the first time. The Joint Commission on Mental Illness and Health publishes findings from hearings conducted between 1955 and 1960, which conclude that state hospitals "are bankrupt beyond remedy" and recommend that community mental health centers be set up to treat those with less severe mental illnesses.

1961   President John F. Kennedy convenes a panel on mental retardation and appoints the Interagency Committee on Mental Health. Two significant publications—Thomas Szasz's *The Myth of Mental Illness* and Erving Goffman's *Asylums*—influence debates about the problems of state asylums and the importance of community-based care.

1962   Ken Kesey's *One Flew over the Cuckoo's Nest* helps turn public opinion against treatments such as electroshock therapy and lobotomy.

1963   President John F. Kennedy signs the Community Mental Health Centers Construction Act, which provides federal funding to create community-based mental health centers.

1965   President Lyndon B. Johnson signs the Social Security Amendments Act of 1965, which creates Medicare and Medicaid.

1966   The first federally funded community mental health center opens. Challenges that seriously mentally ill patients have with taking oral pills according to a schedule lead to the development of the first generation of long-acting injectables (LAIs).

1967   Then California governor Ronald Reagan signs the Lanterman-Petris-Short Act, which limits a family's right to commit a mentally ill relative without due process and reduces the state's institutional expense. The number of mentally ill people in California's criminal justice system doubles within a year.

1971   Senator Edward Kennedy proposes a single-payer health care plan funded through taxes. President Nixon asks for compromises that incorporate private insurance. With union support, Kennedy leaves the deal on the table and walks away. A comprehensive overhaul of health insurance fails. The landmark ruling of *Wyatt v. Stickney* in Alabama sets the precedent that involuntarily hospitalized mental patients have a legal right to adequate treatment.

1972   A Wisconsin court rules in *Lessard v. Schmidt* that involuntary admission to a psychiatric hospital is only permissible if individuals are dangerous to themselves or others.

1973   The Health Maintenance Organization Act promotes the development of health maintenance organizations (HMOs) to control health care costs.

1974   President Nixon proposes a comprehensive health insurance plan that combines private health insurance with state- and federal-supported plans. He later resigns due to the Watergate scandal.

1975   A ruling on *O'Connor v. Donaldson* awards a patient $20,000 in compensatory damages for being kept in a hospital for fifteen years without treatment. Jack Nicholson's portrayal of a mistreated patient in the film version of *One Flew over the Cuckoo's Nest* further turns public opinion against mental hospitals.

1977 By this time, only 650 community mental health centers have been built to serve about 1.9 million patients. Twice the number of community mental health centers are needed. As states close asylums, the deinstitutionalized patients with more serious challenges overwhelm community centers.

1980 President Jimmy Carter signs the Mental Health Systems Act to fund more community mental health centers just a few months before Reagan takes office as president. The act focuses on creating the social conditions for good mental health but lessens the attention given by the federal government to those with the most serious mental illnesses.

1982 A prospective payment system (PPS) for Medicare and Medicaid inpatient services is introduced in Congress, legislated, and implemented by 1983. The intent is to control costs of physical and mental health care.

1986 President Reagan signs the Omnibus Budget Reconciliation Act (OBRA), shifting funding to the state through block grants. The grant process means that community mental health centers compete with other public needs such as housing, food banks, and economic development.

1990 President George H. W. Bush signs the Americans with Disabilities Act (ADA) into law. Throughout the 1990s, private employers and organizations sponsor HMOs, preferred provider organizations (PPOs), and physician-hospital organizations (PHOs) as part of managed care efforts. The FDA approves clozapine to treat the symptoms of schizophrenia, strengthening the prejudice against hospitalization. Wayne Katon, professor of psychiatry at the University of Washington, launches a program that examines the treatment of anxiety and depression in primary care and emphasizes a collaborative care model that later becomes the basis for integrative care.

1993 President Bill Clinton releases the Health Security Plan, the most comprehensive national health insurance plan to be proposed since 1965.

1996 Clinton signs the Health Insurance Portability and Accountability Act (HIPAA), establishing privacy and placing restrictions on how preexisting conditions are treated in group health plans.

1997 The Balanced Budget Act creates the Children's Health Insurance Program (CHIP) and expands Medicaid assistance.

1999 The Supreme Court rules in *Olmstead v. L.C.* that the unjust segregation of people with disabilities violates Title II of the ADA. The case relates to two women with intellectual developmental disabilities and mental illness who were confined to a psychiatric institution even after mental health professionals determined they were capable of moving to a community-based program. Two additional major events include a White House conference on mental health sponsored by Bill Clinton and Tipper Gore and the US Surgeon General's first-ever Report on Mental Health.

2003 President George W. Bush signs the Medicare Prescription Drug, Improvement, and Modernization Act and issues a report from the Commission on Mental Health. The FDA approves the first second-generation LAI, risperidone.

2004 The number of people with serious mental illness grows to about 16 percent of prison and jail inmates (roughly 320,000). In contrast, only about 100,000 psychiatric beds exist in public and private hospitals.

2007 Maine's governor proposes that some county jails be transformed into special facilities for people with mental illness.

2008 The ADA Amendments Act of 2008 (ADAAA) broadens the definition of disability to include people with psychiatric disability and provides legal protections against employment discrimination. The Mental Health Parity and Addiction Equity Act passes and prevents group health plans and health insurance issuers from imposing less favorable benefit limitations on mental health or substance abuse disorder benefits than on medical/surgical benefits.

2009 States cut $4.35 billion in mental health spending in three years due to the Great Recession.

2010 The Affordable Care Act (ACA) passes Congress and mandates
      that insurance companies cover mental health care as one of ten
      essential benefits, including treatment for alcohol, drug, and other
      substance abuse and addiction.

2012 The number of people with serious mental illness being treated
      in jails reaches ten times the number treated in state psychiatric
      hospitals.

2017 President Trump introduces the American Health Care Act
      (AHCA) as a replacement for Obamacare; it passes the House and
      dies in the Senate. The AHCA proposed to reintroduce the ability
      for insurance companies to exclude coverage for some preexisting
      conditions (alcohol and substance abuse, anorexia and bulimia,
      and major depressive and bipolar disorder) and eliminated the
      expansion of Medicaid.

A Tool for Mapping Spaces, Language, and Rituals within Your School, Organization, or Congregation

This book emphasizes the many ways that society contributes to the disablement of people with mental and physical impairments. A variety of tools and inventories have been developed to assist you in mapping spaces, attitudes, language, and rituals within your school, organization, and/or congregation. The questions that follow are offered as a beginning point for examining the presence or absence of people with disabling conditions within schools, organizations, and/or congregational settings. You will want to develop questions to fit your own context. A list of additional tools and inventories to consult is also provided within the "Suggested Readings."

Considering Space

Which places within your school, organization, or congregation are considered the most public, most popular, or most sacred spaces that people gather?

Are there physical barriers to full access for all people in any area? Begin by examining the most public, popular, or sacred spaces and then transition throughout your campus. If full access is not possible, consider what that could potentially convey to people with mobility issues. Are there psychosocial barriers to access these areas?

Where are the spaces that people with physical and mental disabilities are gathering, and what is there to be learned from these spaces?

Are there reserved spaces in your school, organization, or congregation where people experiencing anxiety can find quiet? Is the purpose of these spaces clearly communicated within your school, organization, or congregation?

In addition to focusing on accessible spaces, what else needs to be envisioned in your setting to move toward becoming a community of belonging?

Considering Language

Do people with physical and mental disabilities have the opportunity to name their own conditions within your organization, school, or congregation?

What language is used in classroom documents, lectures, assigned readings, and institutional statements or within services of worship to describe people with various forms of disabling conditions?

How do instructions in group settings (such as classrooms, meetings, or worship) encourage movement and participation? Are participants invited to join in their own ways? Or are there ways that instructions for participation reinforce stigma associated with mental or physical disabilities?

Consider the language used to describe illnesses within your context. Is wholeness referenced only or primarily in relation to the experience of people who are not presently affected by any condition considered disabling? How are stories about healing told? In churches or discussion groups focusing on theology, how is God's reign described through the lens of the embodied realities of people with physical and mental impairments?

Considering Imagery

What types of images are used in the physical space of your institution to represent people with disabilities?

Do the images assume that disabilities are associated with only one circumstance or condition?

How do the images in your physical space portray relationships between people with disabilities and able-bodied, able-minded people? Are there any images of people with disabilities in significant leadership roles?

Considering Content

Are people with physical and mental disabilities not only objects of inquiry within your context but also essential resources for gaining knowledge?

In the case of educational programming, how many classes or study groups focus on disability studies or disability theologies?

Considering Rituals

Do speakers, teachers, or preachers model various forms of embodied participation? For example, are lectures, prayers, or sermons only given from a standing position?

Within a congregation setting, where are the established boundaries of sacred space? What types of images are used within that setting? Are there any images of people with physical and mental impairments?

Considering Your Own Attitudes and Behaviors

In what ways do I contribute to the social process of disablement?

In what ways do I seek to share my own power and privilege in order to contribute to the enablement and empowerment of people with disabilities?

Notes

Introduction

1 National Alliance for Caregiving and the AARP Public Policy Institute, *Caregiving in the U.S. Executive Summary 2015 Report on Family Caregiving*, June 2015, https://tinyurl.com/vfcr78va, 9.

2 National Alliance for Caregiving and the AARP Public Policy Institute, *Caregiving in the U.S. 2020*, May 2020, https://www.caregiving.org/caregiving-in -the-us-2020/, 19.

3 National Alliance on Mental Illness (NAMI) Maryland, *How Siblings and Offspring Deal with Mental Illness*, 2009, https://tinyurl.com/1vqfsio6.

4 Jürgen Moltmann, "God Is Unselfish Love," in *The Emptying God: A Buddhist Christian Conversation*, ed. John B. Cobb Jr. and Christopher Ives (Eugene, OR: Wipf & Stock, 2005), 121.

5 National Alliance for Caregiving and AARP Public Policy Institute, *Caregiving in the U.S. 2020*, 20.

6 Some feminist scholars use the term *patriarchy* (literally meaning "father rule") to name the systems and structures of oppression. Feminist biblical scholar Elisabeth Schüssler-Fiorenza coined the term *kyriarchy* in order "to redefine the analytic category of patriarchy. . . . Kyriarchy is best theorized as a complex pyramidal system of intersecting multiplicative social structures of superordination and subordination, of ruling and oppression." Elisabeth Schüssler-Fiorenza, *Democratizing Biblical Studies: Toward an Emancipatory Educational Space* (Louisville, KY: Westminster John Knox, 2009), 90. The term *kyriarchy* is derived from two Greek words: *kyrios*, meaning "lord," and *archein*, meaning "to rule or dominate."

7 Ellen Ott Marshall, "Bed Rest Stinks," in *Encountering the Sacred: Feminist Reflections on Women's Lives*, ed. Rebecca Todd Peters and Grace Y. Kao (London: T&T Clark, 2019), 34.

8 Marshall, 35.

9 See, for example, Wendy Pyper's study of Canadian women who are caregivers for aging family members. Two-thirds report feeling guilt when they were unable to provide care because of their own need for employment. Pyper, "Aging, Health, and Work," *Perspectives on Labour and Income* 7, no. 2 (February 2006), https://www150.statcan.gc.ca/n1/pub/75-001-x/10206/9095-eng.htm.

10 Valerie Saiving Goldstein, "The Human Situation: A Feminine View," *Journal of Religion* 40, no. 2 (April 1960): 100–112.

11 Alice Walker, *In Search of Our Mother's Gardens: Womanist Prose* (1983; repr., Boston: Mariner, 2003), xii.

12 Irene Oh, "Motherhood in Christianity and Islam: Critiques, Realities, and Possibilities," *Journal of Religious Ethics* 38, no. 4 (December 1, 2010): 638.

13 Isabeth Mendoza, "As Parents and Grandparents Age, More and More Millennials Are Family Caregivers," NPR, March 16, 2019, https://tinyurl.com/4kkxpb2m.

14 Rosemary Radford Ruether, *Many Forms of Madness: A Family's Struggle with Mental Illness and the Mental Health System* (Minneapolis: Fortress, 2010), 26.

15 Ruether, 29.

16 Nancy Fraser, "Crisis of Care? On the Social-Reproductive Contributions of Contemporary Capitalism," in *Social Reproduction Theory: Remapping Class, Recentering Oppression*, ed. Tithi Bhattacharya and Lise Vogel (London: Pluto, 2017), 21–36.

17 "Women Are Well-Represented in Health and Long-Term Care Professions, but Often in Jobs with Poor Working Conditions," OECD, March 2019, https://tinyurl.com/enrv533v.

18 "Women Are Well-Represented."

19 Heidi Hartmann et al., *The Shifting Supply and Demand of Care Work: The Growing Role of People of Color and Immigrants*, Institute for Women's Policy Research report, June 27, 2018, https://tinyurl.com/2z5a2eya.

20 Richard Wilkinson and Kate Pickett, *The Spirit Level: Why Greater Equality Makes Societies Stronger* (New York: Bloomsbury, 2011), 65.

21 "Mental Health by the Numbers," NAMI, last updated March 2021, https://www.nami.org/mhstats.

22 Oren Miron et al., "Suicide Rates among Adolescents and Young Adults in the United States," *Journal of the American Medical Association* 32, no. 23 (2019): 2362–64, https://jamanetwork.com/journals/jama/fullarticle/2735809.

23 Wilkinson and Pickett, *Spirit Level*, 63.

24 NAMI, *Children Mental Health Facts*, September 21, 2016, https://tinyurl.com/3by643xz.

25 Jean M. Twenge, "Increases in Depression, Self-Harm, and Suicide among US Adolescents after 2012 and Links to Technology Use," Psychiatry Online, March 27, 2020, https://prcp.psychiatryonline.org/doi/10.1176/appi.prcp.20190015.

26 Vikram Patel et al., "The *Lancet* Commission on Global Mental Health and Sustainable Development Goals," *Lancet* 392, no. 10157 (October 10, 2018), https://tinyurl.com/6wwfyjsk.

27 Wilkinson and Pickett, *Spirit Level*, 70.

28 Erik Sherman, "America Is the Richest, and Most Unequal, Country," *Fortune*, September 30, 2015, https://tinyurl.com/4qgo8fzq.

29 Additional and more recent research that examines the relationship of religion and mental health is summarized by Harold Koenig in "Research on Religion,

Spirituality, and Mental Health: A Review," *Canadian Journal of Psychiatry* 54, no. 5 (May 2009): 283–91.

30 Adelle Banks, "Preaching on Mental Illness Often Rare, Survey Finds," *Christian Century*, November 12, 2014, 18.

31 R. Abraham, "Mental Illness and the Ministry of the Local Church," *Pastoral Psychology* 63 (2014): 526.

32 Anna Solevåg, *Negotiating the Disabled Body: Representations of Disability in Early Christian Texts* (Atlanta: SBL, 2018), 22.

Part I: Heading into Households and Crawl Spaces

Chapter One: Being Parents and Children in
a Culture of Stigma and Shame

1 Gloria H. Albrecht, "Ideals and Injuries: The Denial of Difference in the Construction of Christian Family Ideals," *Journal of the Society of Christian Ethics* 25, no. 1 (2005): 169.

2 Liza Long, *The Price of Silence: A Mom's Perspective on Mental Illness* (New York: Hudson Street, 2014), 40.

3 Long, 33.

4 Shirley A. Star, "The Public's Ideas about Metal Illness" (paper presented at the annual meeting of the National Association for Mental Health, Indianapolis, IN, November 5, 1955), 6.

5 Star, 34.

6 Stephen Hinshaw, *The Mark of Shame: Stigma of Mental Illness and an Agenda for Change* (Oxford: Oxford University Press, 2007), 34.

7 Hinshaw, 102.

8 Peter Burke, *Brothers and Sisters of Disabled Children* (London: Jessica Kingsley, 2004), 26.

9 Long, *Price of Silence*, 37.

10 Hinshaw, *Mark of Shame*, 13.

11 British Psychological Society, "Society's Critical Response to DSM-V," *Psychologist* 24 (August 2011): 566–69, https://tinyurl.com/2zfd2l4b.

12 Jay Timothy Dolmage, *Disability Rhetoric* (Syracuse: Syracuse University Press, 2014), 6.

13 Mary Jo Iozzio and Miguel J. Romero, "Preface: Engaging Disability," special issue, *Journal of Moral Theology* 6, no. 2 (Fall 2017): 3.

14 R. N. Blick et al., *The Double Burden: Health Disparities among People of Color Living with Disabilities*, Ohio Disability and Health Program, 2015, https://tinyurl.com/y36876dp.

15 See Matt Vasilogambros, "Thousands Lose Right to Vote under 'Incompetence' Laws," Pew Charitable Trust, March 21, 2018, https://tinyurl.com/b5aczzu8; and Kimberly Leonard, "Keeping the 'Mentally Incompetent' from Voting," *Atlantic*, October 17, 2012, https://tinyurl.com/4nytd3uj.

16 "Problems at Home," Association for Children's Mental Health, accessed April 1, 2021, https://tinyurl.com/1tovdy8v.

17 Richard C. Baron and Mark S. Salzer, "Accounting for Unemployment among People with Mental Illness," *Behavioral Sciences and the Law* 20, no. 6 (November 1, 2002): 585.

18 Maria Hengeveld, "Job Hunting with Schizophrenia: Most Americans with the Condition Can and Want to Work. What Is Standing in Their Way?," *Atlantic*, July 28, 2015, https://tinyurl.com/yty82rza.

19 Hengeveld.

20 Mustafa Karakus et al., *Federal Financing of Supported Employment and Customized Employment for People with Mental Illnesses: Final Report*, US Department of Health and Human Services, February 2011, https://tinyurl.com/2vd54tx3, vii.

21 Alison Luciano and Ellen Meara, "The Employment Status of People with Mental Illness: National Survey Data from 2009 and 2010," *Psychiatric Services* 65, no. 10 (October 2014): 1201–9, https://www.ncbi.nlm.nih.gov/pmc/articles/PMC4182106/.

22 "Mental Illness and Violence," *Harvard Mental Health Letter*, January 2011, https://www.health.harvard.edu/newsletter_article/mental-illness-and-violence (URL inactive).

23 See "Mental Health Myths and Facts," MentalHealth.gov, accessed April 7, 2021, https://www.mentalhealth.gov/basics/mental-health-myths-facts; and Sheila A. Schuster, "Don't Use Those with Mental Illness as Scapegoats for Our Nation's Gun Violence Problem," *Courier Journal*, August 23, 2019, https://tinyurl.com/jvbguig7.

24 "Mental Illness and Violence."

25 Emma McGinty et al., "Trends in News Media Coverage of Mental Illness in the United States: 1995–2014," *Health Affairs* 35, no. 6 (June 2016), https://tinyurl.com/ypt5apw8.

26 Michael H. Stone, "Mass Murder, Mental Illness, and Men," *Violence and Gender* 2, no. 1 (March 12, 2015), https://www.liebertpub.com/doi/full/10.1089/vio.2015.0006.

27 Julie Bosman, Kate Taylor, and Tim Arango, "A Common Trait among Mass Killers: Hatred toward Women," *New York Times*, August 10, 2019, https://tinyurl.com/1uqchczr.

28 Camille Gear Rich and Elyn R. Saks, "Introduction: Beating Mental Illness Symposium," *Southern California Interdisciplinary Law Journal* 26 (2016–17): 306, https://heinonline.org/HOL/LandingPage?handle=hein.journals/scid26&div=16&id=&page=.

29 See Treatment Advocacy Center, *Overlooked in the Undercounted: The Role of Mental Illness in Fatal Law Enforcement Encounters*, December 2015, https://tinyurl.com/1avsvkkp.

30 Rebecca Valles, "Disabled behind Bars: The Mass Incarceration of People with Disabilities in America's Jails and Prisons," Center for American Progress, July 18, 2016, https://tinyurl.com/pudm9n6a.

31 Kathleen Gallo, quoted in Patrick W. Corrigan and Petra Kleinlein, "The Impact of Mental Illness Stigma," in *On the Stigma of Mental Illness: Practical Strategies for Research and Social Change*, ed. Patrick Corrigan (2005; repr., Washington, DC: American Psychological Association, 2006), 25.

32 For more information, see Mental Health America's website at https://www .mhanational.org/.

33 E. J. R. David and Anne O. Derthick, "What Is Internalized Oppression and So What?," in *Internalized Oppression: The Psychology of Marginalized Groups*, ed. E. J. R. David (New York: Springer, 2014), 13.

34 Hinshaw, *Mark of Shame*, 6.

35 Ched Myers, "Confronting Legion," Radical Discipleship, June 16, 2016, https://radicaldiscipleship.net/2016/06/16/confronting-legion/.

36 Christine Guth, "Legion No More: Confessions of a Gerasen (Mark 5:1–20)," *Journal of Religion, Disability, and Health* 11, no. 4 (February 21, 2008): 72.

37 Guth, 76.

38 Guth, 72.

39 Researchers describe two aspects of family burden. "Objective burden" refers to the burden that parents, siblings, and partners take on as they invest their time and take on physical care and/or social and financial responsibilities. "Subjective burden" refers to how caregivers perceive of the weight of their responsibilities.

40 Walter Rauschenbusch, *Christianity and the Social Crisis* (Louisville, KY: Westminster John Knox, 1991), 390.

41 Hinshaw, *Mark of Shame*, 108.

42 "Hellish Lives for Children with Severe Mental Illnesses and Their Families, Landmark National Survey Trends," NAMI, July 1, 1999, https://tinyurl.com/ syceq2za.

43 "Hellish Lives."

Chapter Two: Siblings Naming Their Own Experiences

1 Burke, *Brothers and Sisters*, 53.

2 Christopher Griffiths and Jacqueline Sin, "Rethinking Siblings and Mental Illness," *Psychologist* 26, no. 11 (November 1, 2013), https://tinyurl.com/ 36y5d8k9.

3 Jaclyn Leith, Thomas Jewell, and Catherine Stein, "Caregiving Attitudes, Personal Loss, and Related Growth among Siblings of Adults with Mental Illness," *Journal of Child and Family Studies* 27, no. 4 (2018): 1193–1206.

4 Mark Meade, "Merton's Censored Struggle with Suicide," *Merton Journal* 23, no. 2 (Advent 2016): 8–9.

5 Hans Reinders, "Is There Meaning in Disability? Or Is It the Wrong Question?," *Journal of Religion, Disability, and Health* 15, no. 1 (2011): 57.

6 Jenny Gold, "Her Sister's Keeper: Caring for a Sibling with Mental Illness," Kaiser Health News, January 9, 2018, https://tinyurl.com/3u2d65gx.

7 Leith, Jewell, and Stein, "Caregiving Attitudes," 1198.

Part II: History and Current Circumstances

Chapter Three: A Brief Overview of the Treatment of People with Serious Mental Illness in the US Context

1 John Winthrop, "A Model of Christian Charity," in *A Library of American Literature: Early Colonial Literature, 1607–1675*, ed. Edmund Clarence Stedman and Ellen Mackay Hutchinson (New York, 1892), 304–7.

2 Dolmage, *Disability Rhetoric*, 16.

3 Tim Stainton, "Reason's Other: The Emergence of the Disabled Subject in the Northern Renaissance," *Disability and Society* 19, no. 3 (2004): 225–43.

4 Michel Foucault, *Madness and Civilization: A History of Insanity in the Age of Reason* (1965; repr., New York: Vintage, 1988), 7.

5 Foucault, 35.

6 Nicholas Terpstra, *Religious Refugees in the Early Modern World: An Alternative History of the Reformation* (Cambridge: Cambridge University Press, 2015), 21.

7 Susan Sontag, *Illness as Metaphor* (New York: Farrar, Straus and Giroux, 1977), 78.

8 *Oxford English Dictionary*, s.v. "pestilent (*adj.*)," accessed March 27, 2021, https://www.oed.com/.

9 Sherry C. M. Lindquist and Asa Simon Mittman, *Medieval Monsters: Terrors, Aliens, Wonders* (New York: Morgan Library and Museum, 2018), 20.

10 Bettina Bildhauer and Robert Mills, eds., *The Monstrous Middle Ages* (Cardiff: University of Wales Press, 2003), 1.

11 Bildhauer and Mills, 2.

12 Terpstra, *Religious Refugees*, 91.

13 It is worth noting that few cases of "mental maladies" or insanity were recorded among colonists prior to 1700. Historians suggest several reasons for this—for example, colonists would not likely choose to undertake such an arduous journey across the Atlantic with those considered of "unsound mind," and there were relatively few physicians traveling with them and keeping medical records.

14 Cotton Mather, *The Angel of Bethesda: An Essay upon the Common Maladies of Mankind*, ed. Gordon W. Jones (Worcester, MS: American Antiquarian Society and Barre, 1972), 134.

15 Heather Vacek, *Madness: American Protestant Responses to Mental Illness* (Waco, TX: Baylor University Press, 2015), 43.

16 Kenneth J. Weiss, "Isaac Ray's Affair with Phrenology," *Journal of Psychiatry and Law* 34, no. 4 (December 1, 2006): 459.

17 E. Fuller Torrey and Judy Miller, *The Invisible Plague: The Rise of Mental Illness from 1750 to the Present* (New Brunswick, NJ: Rutgers University Press, 2001), 239. In this book, Torrey, a research psychiatrist and mental health advocate, and Miller, a senior research assistant at the Stanley Medical Institution, examine records of insane people in hospitals, jails, prisons, almshouses, and census reports, looking for evidence that insanity was an invisible yet increasing plague across England and Wales, Ireland, Canada, and the United States. The study makes important connections regarding social attitudes toward immigrants, people with mental illness, and people of color.

18 Torrey and Miller, 241.

19 Torrey and Miller, 217.

20 For an excellent discussion of the way cultural expectations are mapped onto extraordinary bodies, read Rosemarie Garland Thomson, "Introduction: From Wonder to Error—a Genealogy of Freak Discourse in Modernity," in *Freakery*, ed. Rosemarie Garland Thomson (New York: New York University Press, 1996).

21 Thomson, 11.

22 Robert Bogdan, "The Social Construction of Freaks," in Thomson, *Freakery*, 23.

23 See Larry Davidson, Jaak Rakfeld, and John Strauss, *The Roots of the Recovery Movement in Psychiatry: Lessons Learned* (West Sussex, UK: John Wiley & Sons, 2010).

24 Davidson, Rakfeld, and Strauss, 9–10.

25 Jay Timothy Dolmage, *Disabled upon Arrival: Eugenics, Immigration, and the Construction of Race and Disability* (Columbus: Ohio State University Press, 2018), 6.

26 Dolmage, 11.

27 Times Special, *Indianapolis Times*, August 14, 1935, 2, Library of Congress, Chronicling of America: Historic Newspapers of America.

28 Christine Rosen, *Preaching Eugenics: Religious Leaders and the American Eugenics Movement* (New York: Oxford University Press, 2004), 16.

29 Vacek, *Madness*, 138.

30 The awarding of a Nobel Peace Prize in Philosophy and Medicine in 1949 to António Egas Moniz (1874–1955), the Portuguese neurologist who developed the lobotomy procedure, speaks to the view at the time that the procedure held great promise. Today, the Nobel Prize given for the lobotomy procedure is considered among the worst decisions made by the Nobel Foundation.

31 Joel Braslow, *Mental Ills and Bodily Cures: Psychiatric Treatment in the First Half of the Twentieth Century* (Berkeley: University of California Press, 1997), 166.

32 As quoted in Vacek, *Madness*, 115.

33 Vacek, 15.

34 Glenn H. Asquith Jr., ed., *Vision from a Little Known Country: A Boisen Reader* (Decatur, GA: Journal of Pastoral Care Publications, 1992), 9.

35 Anton T. Boisen, "Cooperative Inquiry in Religion" (1945), in Asquith, *Vision*, 82.

36 Anton T. Boisen, "Concerning the Relationship between Religious Experience and Mental Disorders" (1923), in Asquith, *Vision*, 18.

37 Vacek, *Madness*, 123.

38 Albert Q. Maisel, "Bedlam 1946," *Life Magazine*, May 6, 1946, https://www.pbs.org/wgbh/americanexperience/features/lobotomist-bedlam-1946/.

39 See the "Timeline of Significant Events Related to Policy Shifts, Treatment, and Attitudes toward Mental Illness from the Mid-twentieth Century to the Present" in this book. Noteworthy efforts prior to the 1980s included First Lady Betty Ford's open support of mental health care, Senator Edward Kennedy's and President Richard Nixon's work to advance a comprehensive health insurance plan, and President Jimmy and First Lady Rosalyn Carter's support of the Mental Health Systems Act.

Chapter Four: Prescription for Poverty

1 "Mental Health, Poverty, and Development," World Health Organization, March 27, 2021, https://tinyurl.com/1lkhcviu.

2 "Serious Mental Illness among Adults below the Poverty Line," Substance Abuse and Mental Health Services Administration (SAMHSA), March 30, 2021, https://tinyurl.com/3psymfhe.

3 "How Is Poverty Status Related to Disability?," Center for Poverty and Inequality, University of California, Davis, March 30, 2021, https://tinyurl.com/aca5k8pe.

4 Jill Quadagno, "Why the U.S. Has No National Health Insurance: Stakeholder Mobilization against the Welfare State, 1945–1996," *Journal of Health and Social Behavior* 45, extra issue (2004): 25.

5 Liz Essley Whyte, "State Policies May Send People with Disabilities to the Back of the Line for Ventilators," Center for Public Integrity, April 8, 2020, https://tinyurl.com/4uc53kzs.

6 E. F. Torrey notes that in 1998, the *Chicago Tribune* published a series on the increase of mentally ill patients in state nursing homes and reported that often, the organizations modified patient files and diagnoses so that they could gain access to Medicaid dollars. Torrey, *American Psychosis: How the Federal Government Destroyed the Mental Illness Treatment System* (Oxford: Oxford University Press, 2014), EBSCOhost e-book collection.

7 Stephen Melek, Daniel Perlman, and Stoddard Davenport, *Addiction and Mental Health vs. Physical Health: Analyzing Disparities in Network Use and Provider Reimbursement Rates*, Milliman Research Report, December 2017, https://tinyurl.com/dpevthnx.

8   Cynthia Koons and John Tozzi, "As Suicides Rise, Insurers Find Ways to Deny Mental Health Coverage," *Bloomberg Businessweek*, May 16, 2019, https://tinyurl.com/wpb6f9ur.

9   Scott Simon, "Kentucky Gov. Matt Bevin on Requiring Medicaid Recipients to Work," NPR, January 13, 2018, https://tinyurl.com/cypv5ntf.

10 Sharon V. Betcher, *Spirit and the Politics of Disablement* (Minneapolis: Fortress, 2007), 14.

11 "How Much to Earn to Qualify," Disability Benefits Help, March 25, 2021, https://tinyurl.com/4unkbhrh.

12 Hengeveld, "Job Hunting with Schizophrenia."

13 E. F. Torrey et al., "The Treatment of Persons with Mental Illness in Prisons and Jails: A State Survey," Treatment Advocacy Center, April 8, 2014, https://tinyurl.com/9hwue9p7.

14 See Luona Lin, Karen Stamm, and Peggy Christidis, "How Diverse Is the Psychology Workforce?," *Monitor on Psychology* 49, no. 2 (February 2018): 19, https://tinyurl.com/3co6zpdh.

15 "State Mental Health Agency (SMHA) per Capita Mental Health Services Expenditures," Kaiser Family Foundation, 2013, https://tinyurl.com/1k3dmebi.

16 K. Bryant Smalley, Jacob C. Warren, and Jackson P. Rainer, eds., *Rural Mental Health: Issues, Policies, and Best Practices* (New York: Springer, 2012), 5.

17 Mary Gerisch, "Health Care as a Human Right." April 19, 2021. https://tinyurl.com/4rddz9ds.

18 See "Mental Health and Development," United Nations, last updated August 29, 2017, https://tinyurl.com/4963vj8b.

Part III: Empowerment, Alternatives, and Advocacy

Chapter Five: Biblical Threads of Empowerment

1   Robert Garland, *The Eye of the Beholder: Deformity and Disability in the Graeco-Roman World* (Ithaca, NY: Cornell University Press, 1995), 8.

2   Dolmage, *Disability Rhetoric*, 64.

3   Garland, *Eye of the Beholder*, 1.

4   Garland, 31.

5   Martha L. Rose, *The Staff of Oedipus: Transforming Disability in Ancient Greece* (Ann Arbor: University of Michigan Press, 2003), 2.

6   Rose, 50–65.

7   Solevåg, *Negotiating the Disabled Body*, 22.

8   Aristotle, *The History of Animals*, trans. D'Arcy Wentworth Thompson (n.p.: Infomations, 2000), 10, ProQuest.

9   Pieter van der Horst, "Organized Charity in the Ancient World: Pagan, Jewish, Christian," *Jewish and Christian Communal Identities in the Roman World* 94 (January 2016): 117.

10 Pieter van der Horst, "How the Poor Became Blessed," *Aeon*, March 28, 2021, https://aeon.co/essays/the-poor-might-have-always-been-with-us-but-charity -has-not.

11 Solevåg, *Negotiating the Disabled Body*, 37.

12 See Cicero, *De officiis* 2.15.54; Seneca, *De vita beata* 23–24; A. R. Hands, *Charities and Social Aid in Greece and Rome* (Ithaca, NY: Cornell University Press, 1968), 64–76.

13 Margaret Aymer, "Horizons Bible Study Lesson: Matthew 5:6; Luke 6:21a, 25a; Psalm 107:1–9," *Unbound: An Interactive Journal of Christian Social Justice* (February/March 2012), https://tinyurl.com/ye9e2nmv.

14 Gregory Mobley, *The Return of the Chaos Monsters—and Other Backstories of the Bible* (Grand Rapids, MI: Eerdmans, 2012), 2.

15 Mobley, 14.

16 See Mary Douglas, *Purity and Danger: An Analysis of Concepts of Pollution and Taboo*, vol. 2, *Mary Douglas Collected Works* (1966; repr., New York: Routledge, 2003).

17 Amos Yong, *Theology and Down Syndrome: Reimagining Disability in Late Modernity* (Waco, TX: Baylor University Press, 2007), 23.

18 Gregory Lamb, "Sinfully Stereotyped: Jesus's Desire to Correct Ancient Physiognomic Assumptions in the Gospel according to Luke," *Word and World* 37, no. 2 (Spring 2017): 179.

19 The term *skolops* is also used in the Septuagint in Numbers (33:55), Hosea (2:6), and Ezekiel (28:24) and describes thorns in all three of those books.

20 See Mikeal C. Parsons, *Body and Character in Luke and Acts: The Subversion of Physiognomy in Early Christianity* (Waco, TX: Baylor University Press, 2011), 48–49.

21 See Beverly Roberts Gaventa, *Our Mother St. Paul* (Louisville, KY: Westminster John Knox, 2007).

Chapter Six: Communities of Empowerment and Belonging

1 Hildegard of Bingen, *Holistic Healing*, ed. Mary Palmquist and John Kulas, trans. Manfred Pawlik, Patrick Madigan, and John Kulas (Collegeville, MN: Liturgical, 1994), 46–47.

2 Even today, exorcism is seen as a form of charity thought to benefit people who "suffer" from mental illness. See Chris French, "Pope Francis and the Psychology of Exorcism and Possession," *Guardian*, July 9, 2014, https://tinyurl.com/b7majey6.

3 Hildegard, *Holistic Healing*, 46–47.

4 Reggie Williams, "Developing a Theologia Crucis: Dietrich Bonhoeffer in the Harlem Renaissance," *Theology Today* 71, no. 1 (2014): 46.

5 Bernd Wannenwetsch, "'My Strength Is Made Perfect in Weakness': Bonhoeffer and the War over Disabled Life," in Brian Brock and John Swinton, *Disability*

in the Christian Tradition: A Reader (Grand Rapids, MI: Eerdmans, 2012), 371.

6 Wannenwetsch, 365.

7 Wannenwetsch, 374.

8 Lulu Miller, "The Problem with the Solution," *Invisibilia*, NPR, July 1, 2016, https://tinyurl.com/yds8u42n.

9 Jason Reimer Greig, *Reconsidering Intellectual Disability: L'Arche, Medical Ethics, and Christian Friendship* (Washington, DC: Georgetown University Press, 2015), 3.

10 Greig, 4.

11 Grieg, 128.

12 Hans S. Reinders, "Being with the Disabled: Jean Vanier's Theological Realism," in Brock and Swinton, *Disability in the Christian Tradition*, 492.

Chapter Seven: Cultivating Belonging and Practicing Intentional Prayer and Advocacy

1 John Swinton, "From Inclusion to Belonging: A Practical Theology of Community, Disability, and Humanness," *Journal of Religion, Disability, and Health* 16, no. 2 (2012): 173.

2 Swinton, 181.

3 Jason Whitehead, "Ghosts and Guests: A Pastoral Theology of Belonging for Ministry with Persons with Mental Illness," *Journal of Pastoral Care and Counseling* 70, no. 4 (2016): 260.

4 I think the writings of theorists such as Edward Said, Gayatri Spivak, and Frantz Fanon can be helpful here in understanding the indelible psychological imprint stigma leaves on people with serious mental illness and their families. Said is a postcolonial theorist who writes about the experience of Palestinian people living in Israel. He argues that the values of the colonizer are internalized by the colonizer as well as the victim of conquest. People in a superior position may accept "their almost metaphysical obligation to rule subordinate, inferior, or less advanced people" and those who are considered inferior internalize the stigma and their status. Edward Said, *Culture and Imperialism* (London: Chatto & Windus, 1993), 10.

5 McGinty et al., "Trends in News Media."

6 Andrew Whitehead, "Religion and Disability: Variation in Religious Service Attendance Rates for Children with Chronic Health Conditions," *Journal for the Scientific Study of Religion* 57, no. 2 (June 1, 2018): 378.

7 See E. W. Carter et al., "Congregational Participation of a National Sample of Adults with Intellectual and Developmental Disabilities," *Intellectual and Developmental Disabilities* 53, no. 6 (2015): 381–93.

8 See "U.S. Congregational Life Survey," Association of Religion Data Archives, 2001, https://tinyurl.com/4afsbs9c.

9   *Study of Acute Mental Illness and Christian Faith: Research Report*, Lifeway Research, 2014, https://tinyurl.com/6tje386z.

10 Ian Lovett, "'It's like I Got Kicked Out of My Family': Churches Struggle with Mental Health in the Ranks," *Wall Street Journal*, January 20, 2020, https://tinyurl.com/23bnxtk4.

11 Naomi Annandale and Erik Carter, "Disability and Theological Education: A North American Study," *Theological Education* 48, no. 2 (2014): 83–102.

12 Examples include the Center for Disability and Ministry at Western Theological Seminary (https://tinyurl.com/1ezn2icu) and the Summer Institute on Theology and Disability (https://tinyurl.com/15fxdeo0).

13 Rebecca F. Spurrier, *The Disabled Church: Human Difference and the Art of Communal Worship* (New York: Fordham University Press, 2019), 15.

14 Spurrier, 60.

15 Spurrier, 60.

16 Whitehead, "Ghosts and Guests," 261.

17 William Gaventa, "Preaching Disability: The Whole of Christ's Body in Word and Practice," *Review and Expositor* 113, no. 2 (2016): 226.

18 Erik W. Carter, "A Place of Belonging: Research at the Intersection of Faith and Disability," *Review and Expositor* 113, no. 2 (May 2016): 172.

19 Spurrier, *Disabled Church*, 133.

20 Spurrier, 132.

21 See Debra McKinney, "Listening Post Is 'Here to Be Present and Loving,'" *Anchorage Daily News*, October 2, 2009, https://tinyurl.com/v898a3ie; and the Sidewalk-Talk website at https://www.sidewalk-talk.org/.

22 Whitehead, "Religion and Disability," 379.

23 Connie Larkman, "Pennsylvania Congregation's Pet Therapy Program Is Perfect: 3 Great Loves Ministry," United Church of Christ, March 13, 2018, https://tinyurl.com/4ns2b5wx.

24 Sarah Griffith Lund, *Blessed are the Crazy: Breaking the Silence about Mental Illness, Family, Church*. St. Louis: Chalice Press, 2014, 51.

25 Kathy Black, *A Healing Homiletic: Preaching and Disability* (Nashville: Abingdon, 1996), 177.

26 Black, 179.

27 Black, 36.

28 Carter, "Place of Belonging," 174.

29 See Matthew Green, "Coronavirus: How These Disabled Activists Are Taking Matters into Their Own (Sanitized) Hands," KQED, March 17, 2020, https://tinyurl.com/183079ay.

30 Dana Dillon, "The Vital Cell: Subsidiarity and a Family-Centered Approach to Accompanying Persons with Mental Illness" (paper submitted to 2020 College Theology Society Annual Volume, July 1, 2020), http://www.collegetheology.org/Ethics-Session-4.

31 Dillon.

32 Carter, "Place of Belonging," 177.

33 Ramón Luzárraga, "Accompaniment with the Sick: An Authentic Christian Vocation That Rejects the Fallacy of Prosperity Theology," *Journal of Moral Theology* 8, no. 1 (January 1, 2019): 77–88.

34 Craig Rennebohm with David Paul, *Souls in the Hands of a Tender God: Stories of the Search for Home and Healing on the Streets* (Boston: Beacon, 2008), 136.

35 Carter, "Place of Belonging," 177.

36 Carter, 178.

37 Francisco Argüelles Paz y Puente, "'We Are Never Alone': Some Thought on Accompaniment Communities," *Comment Magazine*, 2019, https://tinyurl.com/y9p38p4u.

38 Paz y Puente, 58–59.

39 Paz y Puente, 60.

Suggested Readings

A variety of resources are easily accessible and available for free download online. See the following sample of denominational and interfaith statements and other sources related to mental and physical disabilities.

Publications

American Association of People with Disabilities (AAPD) and Interfaith Advocacy Coalition. *That All May Worship: An Interfaith Welcome to People with Disabilities*. Accessed March 31, 2021. https://www.aapd.com/publications/that-all-may-worship-2/.

American Baptist Home Mission Society. "Communities of Care: The Church and Mental Illness." *Christian Citizen* 2 (2014). https://network.crcna.org/disability-concerns/communities-care-church-and-mental-illness.

Communitas Supportive Care Society. *God of All Comfort: Mental Health Resources for Church Worship*. 2018. https://www.communitascare.com/stories/worship-resource-updated/.

Evangelical Lutheran Church in America. *The Body of Christ and Mental Illness*. Chicago: Evangelical Lutheran Church in America, 2012. https://tinyurl.com/y64tu9rk.

Intelligent Design Exposed. "United Methodist Church: An Apology for Support of Eugenics." idexposed, May 19, 2008. https://tinyurl.com/e24fsv2n.

Presbyterian Church USA. *Comfort My People: A Policy Statement on Serious Mental Illness.* Louisville, KY: Presbyterian Church USA, 2008. https://www.pcusa.org/resource/comfort-my-people-policty-statement-serious-mental/.

United Church of Christ. "Disabilities and Mental Health Justice." Accessed April 7, 2021. https://tinyurl.com/4ym95a7s.

United Church of Christ Disabilities Ministries. *Any Body, Every Body, Christ's Body: A Guide for Congregations, Associations, and Conferences for Becoming Accessible to All.* Spring 2016. https://uccdm.org/a2a/a2a-guide/.

Websites

The Interfaith Network on Mental Illness provides online resources related to the needs of different faith traditions and promotes a national weekend of prayer for Faith.Hope.Life. You can access their website online at https://theactionalliance.org/faith-hope-life/interfaith-network-mental-illness.

NAMI FaithNet has a variety of resources available at https://www.nami.org/Get-Involved/NAMI-FaithNet.

The National Catholic Partnership on Disability provides a variety of resources for individuals, parishes, priests, families, and schools on their website at https://ncpd.org/.

Pathways to Promise is an interfaith cooperative that provides resources, training, and consultation for faith groups wanting to develop ministries with and for people with serious mental illness and their families. You can find more information on their website at https://www.pathways2promise.org/.

The United Church of Christ Mental Health Network offers a variety of resources that promote inclusion and can help congregations work together to eliminate the stigma associated with serious mental illness. You can find these resources at https://www.mhn-ucc.org/.

Index